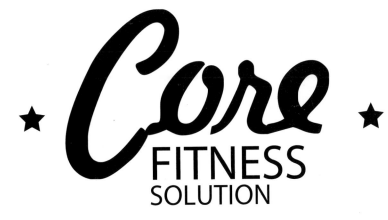

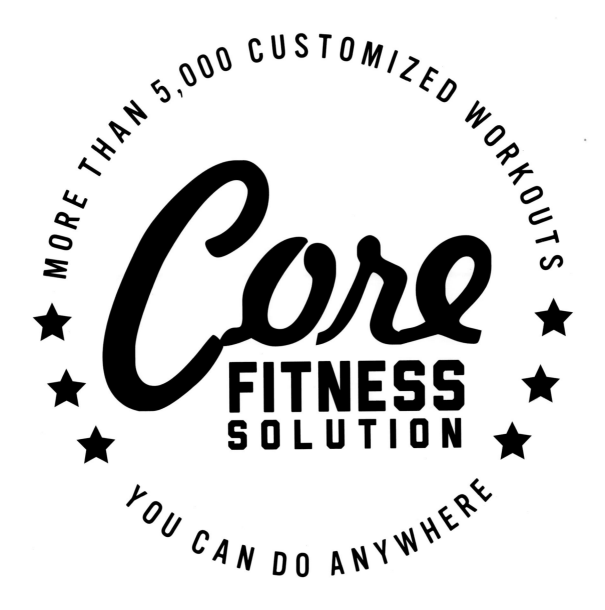

MORE THAN 5,000 CUSTOMIZED WORKOUTS

Core

FITNESS
SOLUTION

YOU CAN DO ANYWHERE

MICHAEL DE MEDEIROS +
KENDALL WOOD. NASM. "KING OF ABS"
PHOTOGRAPHY BY ROBERT REIFF

Fair Winds Press
100 Cummings Center, Suite 406L
Beverly, MA 01915

fairwindspress.com • bodymindbeautyhealth.com

© 2014 Fair Winds Press

First published in the USA in 2014 by
Fair Winds Press, a member of
Quarto Publishing Group USA Inc
100 Cummings Center
Suite 406-L
Beverly, MA 01915-6101
www.fairwindspress.com
Visit www.bodymindbeautyhealth.
com. It's your personal guide to a happy,
healthy, and extraordinary life!

18 17 16 15 14   1 2 3 4 5

ISBN: 978-1-59233-640-1

Digital edition published in 2014
eISBN: 978-1-62788-184-5

Library of Congress Cataloging-in-
Publication Data available

Cover design by Burge Agency
Book design by Burge Agency
Artwork by Pete Usher
Photography by Robert Reiff

Printed and bound in China

The information in this book is for
educational purposes only. It is not
intended to replace the advice of a
physician or medical practitioner. Please
see your health care provider before
beginning any new health program.

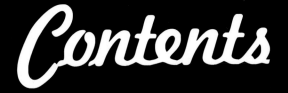

Contents

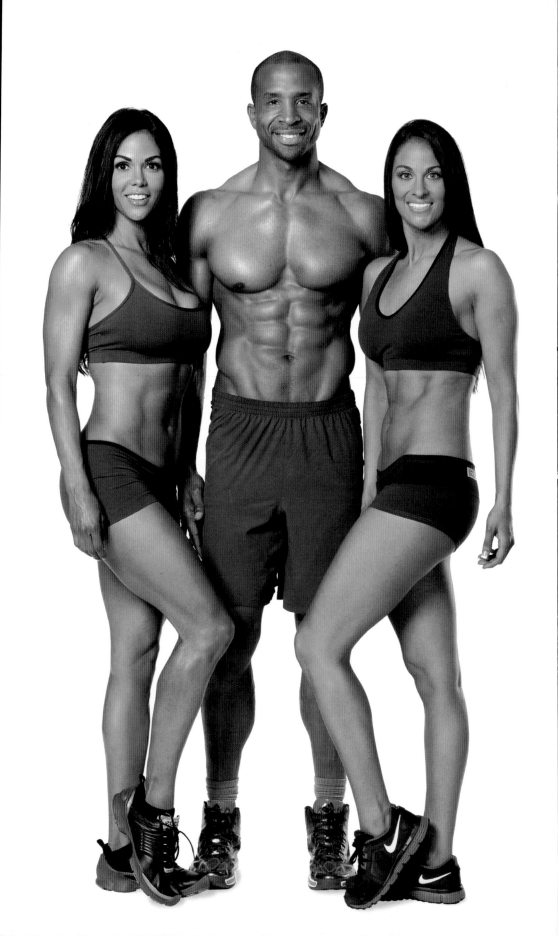

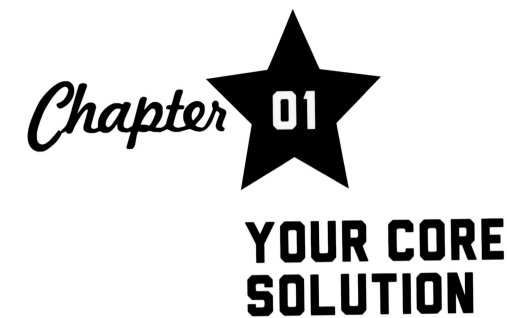

Chapter 01

YOUR CORE SOLUTION

SIX-PACK ABS! LOSE YOUR GUT! BLAST BELLY FAT! FLAT ABS FAST! WHITTLE YOUR MIDDLE! GET ABS IN MINUTES! BUILD A SEXY WAIST! GET AN EIGHT-PACK! SLICED ABS IN ONE WORKOUT!

You won't be seeing any of these promises in this book. Why? Because, by purchasing this book you've made a decision that mere promises aren't what you're looking for. A complicated workout with dozens of exercises hasn't worked for you. That fitness gadget you bought off an infomercial earned its spot in your garage between your tangled Christmas lights and old VCR. The meal plan you downloaded that promised instant health made you sick. Your gym membership does little more than keep your library card company in the last slot of your wallet. You've been through the promises. What you want is a solution.

But before you think you found another easy answer, take note: There is no single solution that works for everyone. The answer is a custom solution just for you. But you're the only person who can create that solution.

A magazine can't do it. A product off of late-night television can't do it. Ultimately, even a meal plan and workout are only as effective as the effort you put into them. They, too, are fundamentally flawed because they are made to suit the masses—they simply aren't made specifically for you. Even a personal trainer can only react to what you're willing to divulge and, let's face it: Nobody's totally honest with trainers or nutritionists. The only honest conversation you can have when it comes to your appearance, your health and your fitness happens when you're being honest with yourself. Bottom line: The only real solution that will yield results can only come from you.

The last time you were at the gym, someone told you to do four sets of 12 repetitions of a certain exercise. It may have been something you read, something you were told, or something you saw someone else do. Nobody ever said why. You weren't told what weight to use for each contraction. You just followed the orders that were given, didn't you? But only you knew when your muscles started to burn. Only you knew what weight was comfortable, what weight was too much, and what weight was pointless to try. Why? Because only you know your body, your commitment to being healthy and the effort you're willing to apply in your quest to achieve it.

That's why *Core Fitness Solution* is different from any other fitness plan you've read, heard about or tried. This really is *your* workout—you design it, you do the work, you decide the intensity, and you see the results. But results come best when you're fully prepared. Before making your workouts, you need to understand the core, its importance and how it affects nearly every movement you make as an athlete, a weekend warrior, or an everyday person.

UNDERSTANDING YOUR CORE

If you fall prey to the vernacular found in most much-hyped gadgets, books, and magazine articles, you'll fall for the half-truth that your core is composed of the six abdominal muscles that seemingly only fitness models ever have. The elusive six-pack is actually made up of one muscle called the rectus abdominis. The appearance of the six distinct muscles comes from connective tissue. The muscles on the sides are called the obliques. While abs are definitely a vital element of your core, the truth is your core is the full circumference of your midsection. Think of it as the middle of your body. The middle, of course, isn't just on the front of your torso; it's also on your back and sides. That middle is integral to every step, move, push, pull and stretch you do every day. *That* is your core. Ultimately, you need to think of your core as the engine in a car: It is responsible for every motion, fast or slow, precise or relaxed, not just looking good.

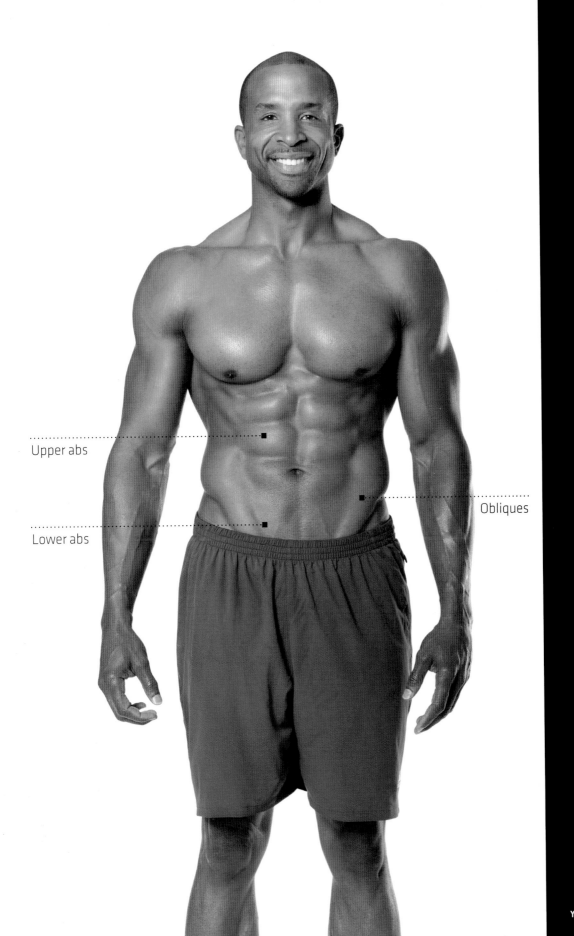

Upper abs

Lower abs

Obliques

Just because there are muscle targets mentioned in this book, don't think that you can simply isolate a specific segment of your abs and solely target-train them. Sure, you can emphasize certain areas with certain moves, but if you already have upper abs and want to just train your lower abs, you're not using this book correctly. Please refer to the next section for more direction.

While most other workouts will focus on the aesthetically pleasing muscles in the front, any athlete will tell you without hesitation that a strong core beats ripped abs any day. The best part of Core Fitness Solution, however, is that while we're helping you build the core you need, we're also making sure your abs pop just as noticeably as any avid gym-goer—only you won't be spending long hours in the gym to do it!

HOW TO USE *CORE FITNESS SOLUTION*

The following chapters titled "Lower Abs," "Upper Abs," "Obliques," and "Total Core" are composed of the best exercises for each specific target mentioned. Within each chapter you'll find detailed descriptions of each move, intensity tips, beginner's advice, and additional information on how to get the most out of your core workouts. We've designed the plan to be as easy to use as possible—while maintaining the promise that you decide your workout. With that said, there are only two rules to follow:

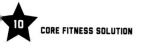

1. Each workout you create must consist of two exercises from each chapter. That means every workout will have eight exercises in total. No more, no less! Because you'll be hitting every angle of your core throughout this process, all the typical complications of other workout plans are totally washed away.

2. Each exercise must be done to failure. That means you'll be doing eight exercises until you simply can't do them anymore. If you can do a couple of exercises 22 times each, but can only get to 12 on the rest, that's fine. As a general rule, you should try to hit 12 to 24 reps in each set. If you find yourself consistently only managing a few reps on a specific move, you should probably try an easier variation. By the same

token, if you're doing 50 reps of the same move every time you do it, it's time to graduate to a more advanced move. If you're performing timed exercises, then stay with 15 to 60 seconds; if this is too easy, you'll need to select a more advanced move.

Ultimately, the choice is yours and is based on your effort, fitness level, and desired workout intensity. We suggest recording your reps in the training log in chapter 7 to track your progress. The goal here is to work your way up through the beginner and intermediate moves to the advanced moves. This ensures that you build strength through repetitions and gradually add more intense moves. It also reduces the risk of injury that is caused by performing the wrong moves for your fitness level.

Each exercise in this book has a beginner and an advanced version for this purpose. Be honest with yourself and your selections. Core strength and visible abs will come more quickly than you think.

Because the core is in constant use, there's little fear of overworking the area as you would with your other major muscle groups. As such, you can do a customized *Core Fitness Solution* workout every day if you wish, or you can do them on off days from your full-body workouts or in conjunction with them. The choice is yours! You can also do more than one workout each day, though we do not advise more than two on any single day. Since you should be working to failure on each move, one workout each day should suffice.

MORE THAN 5,000 WORKOUTS?

Sound like an unbelievable promise? Think again. The entire premise of this book is based on you creating your own daily workouts, and although there are very few rules you have to follow, the few that you do are set in stone. By selecting two exercises from each category of exercises in this book—upper abs, lower abs, obliques, and total core—you're creating a specific workout plan for your day. There are 12 exercises in upper abs, 10 in lower abs, 12 in obliques and 19 in total core. We consulted with two colleges to calculate the exact amount of workouts in this book and they both agreed on 63,577,800 total possible configurations from these options. If we hear anyone complaining that there aren't enough options in this book, we'll find you and hurl more than sixty-three million sweaty gym socks at you!

Use the Core Fitness Solution Checklist, on pages 13–15, to quickly and easily design your workouts. It lists all 53 exercises described in the book, organizes them by category, and even provides a thumbnail to help you quickly recall the exercises you love—and the ones you love to hate.

CORE FITNESS SOLUTION EXERCISE CHECKLIST

CH. 2 LOWER ABS

1. Pelvic Tilt

2. Ab Crunch with Vertical Legs

3. U-Boat

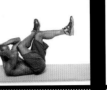

4. Figure Four Leg Raise and Crunch

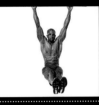

5. Captain's Chair Leg Lift

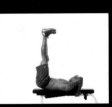

6. Hanging Leg Raise

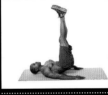

7. Flutter Kicks

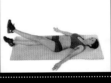

8. Vertical Leg Crunch

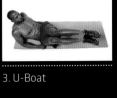

9. Bench Leg Raise

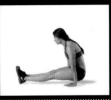

10. Reclining Leg Circles

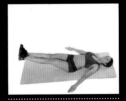

11. Hover

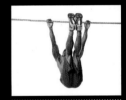

12. Toes to Bar Hanging Leg Raise

CH. 3 UPPER ABS

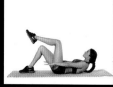

1. Crunch and Reach

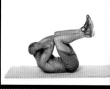

2. Dead Bug

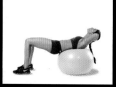

3. Stability Ball Crunch

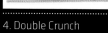
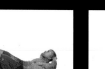

4. Double Crunch

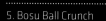

5. Bosu Ball Crunch

6. Leg Climb

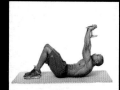
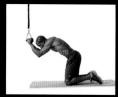

7. Weighted Crunch

8. Kneeling Resistance Band Crunch

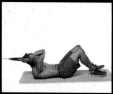
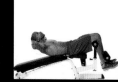

9. Cable Crunch

10. Decline Bench Curl

CH. 4 OBLIQUES

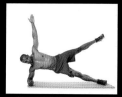
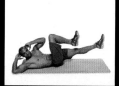

1. Side Plank

2. Side Bend

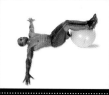
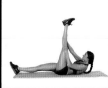

3. Stability Ball Hip Rolls

4. Bicycle Crunch

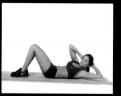
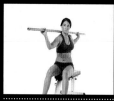

5. Cross Body Crunch

6. Seated Broom Twist

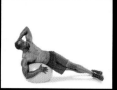
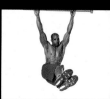

7. Stability Ball Oblique Crunch

8. Hanging Leg Raises with Twists

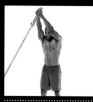
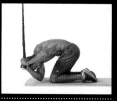

9. Landmines

10. Kneeling Cable Oblique Crunch

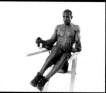
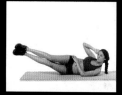

11. Captain's Chair Side Leg Lift

12. Oblique Crunch with Legs Up

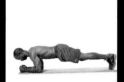
1. Plank

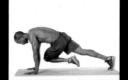
2. Spidermans

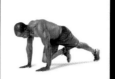
3. Mountain Climbers

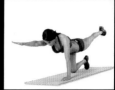
4. Dog Pointers

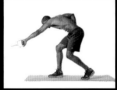
5. Roll-Ups

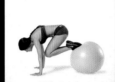
6. Stability Ball Knee Tuck

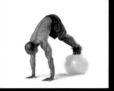
7. Pike

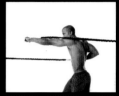
8. Cable Push-Pull

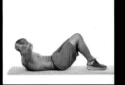
9. Cable Lawnmower

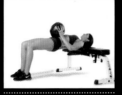
10. Weighted Hip Raise on a Bench

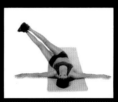
11. Windshield Wipers

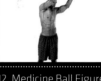
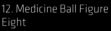
12. Medicine Ball Figure Eight

13. Medicine Ball Wood Chopper

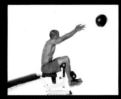
14. Decline Medicine Ball Toss

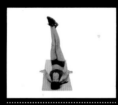
15. Corkscrew

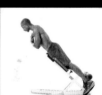
16. Reverse Hyperextensions

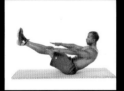
17. Isometric V-Hold

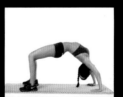
18. Jump Squat with Twist

19. Bridge

CORE STRESS TEST

Before jumping into any serious workout plan, you should consult a physician. You should also test your fitness level before deciding the intensity of your workouts. This section of *Core Fitness Solution* is your test to see how fit your core is before you begin your custom workouts, and then to see how far you've come after progressing through your training.

Why do you need to test your core strength before doing these workouts? Well, the truth is that you actually don't have to, but we recommend it for several reasons. In our years of helping people with their fitness and health, one thing has always been constant: Left unchecked, or untested, people will almost always jump into a workout plan that is far above their capacity. This results in injury that keeps people away from the gym, ruining any efforts or desires they had on improving their lives. Testing your fitness level before starting a program will also help you better select your workouts and track your progress.

With that in mind, we've devised a test that measures your stability, endurance, and overall core strength. The test is based on one exercise: the plank. Execution of the move is simple, but becomes more and more challenging with each passing second.

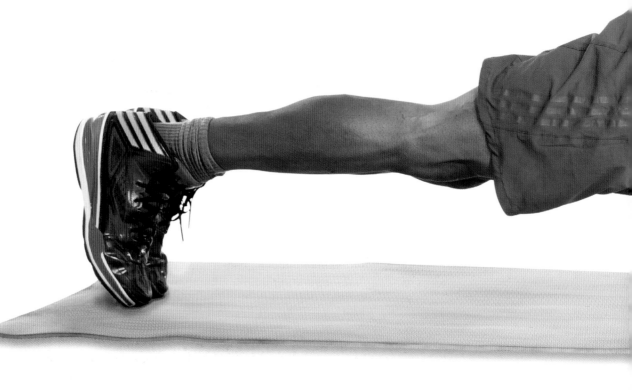

THE PLANK

Lie face down on a mat so your toes, forearms, and fists are holding all of your weight off the ground. Your body should create a straight, plank-like line. Create a neutral (flat) spine by tilting your pelvis forward. Engage your abdominals, glutes, and thigh muscles. Your butt and hips should stay in this same line; make sure they don't sag or rise beyond the level. Do not round your shoulders. Maintain this position throughout while looking straight down at your hands.

Depending on your workout philosophy, you could hold this move to failure once or several times (which is what we suggest) or you could hold it for a set time span and repeat the interval as many times as you like (much like you would with reps). For the purpose of this test, you'll be staying in the plank as long as you can, but, to better test your overall core strength, endurance, and stability, we've added intensifiers, target-specific variations, and intervals.

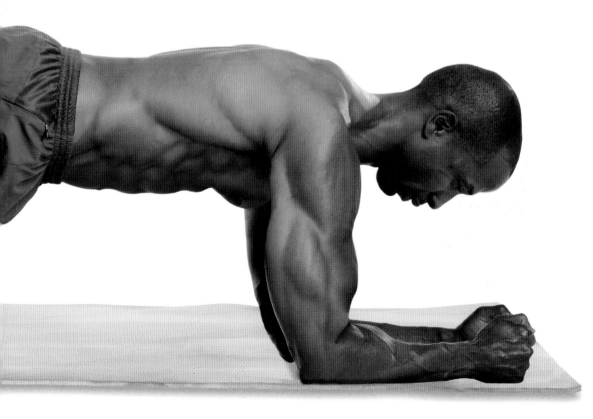

PLANK VARIATIONS

There are several variations to the basic plank exercise. In order to fully test your core strength, we have incorporated the ones we feel are the best gauges to understanding your fitness level. Here is a brief description of each one found in the test that follows.

Plank with arm raise: From the basic plank position previously described, raise one arm off the floor so your fingers are pointing straight ahead with your palm facing inward. Your arm should not go above your shoulders, which must maintain a straight line with your body.

Plank with leg raise: Lift one leg off the ground so it creates a parallel line with the floor. Keep the leg straight with no bend in your knee and point your toes away.

Plank with leg and arm raise: Raise your left leg and right arm together (as described) and then your left arm and right leg together.

Plank with leg and arm raise

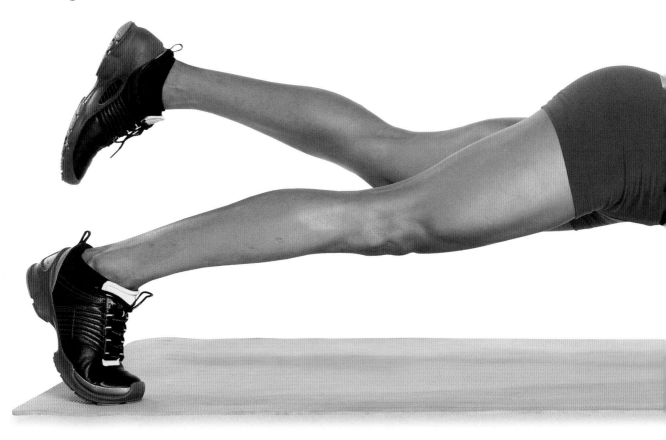

Plank with leg and arm raise with crunch: As previously described, raise alternating legs and arms, but before returning to the plank position, crunch your leg (with bended knee) and arm (with bended elbow) into your torso and hold for one count.

Side plank: Balance yourself so only your left foot and left forearm and fist are holding all your weight.

Side plank with hip raise: Perform the side plank as already described, but lower your hip to the floor and then raise your hip back to the side plank position.

Side plank with front leg drive: Perform the side plank as previously described, and drive the knee of your top leg toward your chest, forming a right angle at the hip and abdominal area.

Side plank with double leg drive: This is the same as above but with both legs.

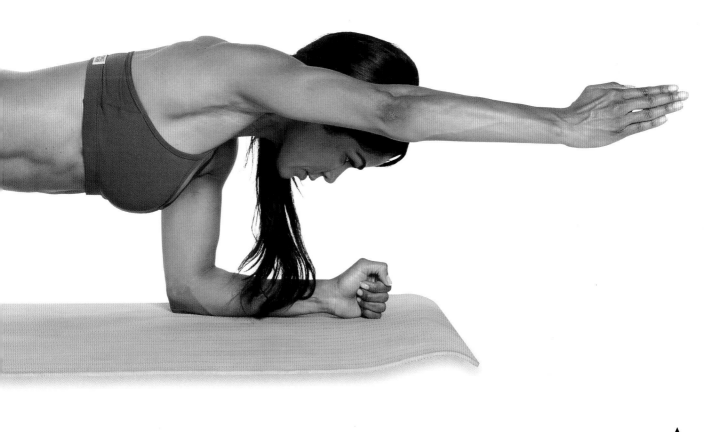

THE TEST

As you can see from the chart that follows, the test is broken down into timed intervals. You are not to rest between intervals or performance levels. This is a running clock test. We suggest a training partner time you, or that you follow your own progress on a device placed between your fists. Each interval is a specific form of the plank and the further you get into the test, the better your core strength, endurance, and stability.

Where you've placed on the chart dictates where you should begin your training in this book. If you've fallen in the Beginner or Intermediate sections, you should start your exercises with the beginner's tips. If you're in the Average or Advanced sections, perform the moves pictured and described in each chapter. If you've scored in the Superior or Elite sections, challenge yourself with the advanced tips.

We recommend coming back to this test every 30 days so you can measure your progress in your core performance training.

BRACKET 1: Beginner

Plank	10 seconds
Raise arm	5 seconds each arm
Raise leg	5 seconds each leg
Side plank (stacked feet)	10 seconds each side

BRACKET 2: Intermediate

Plank	20 seconds
Raise left arm and right leg	10 seconds
Raise right arm and left leg	10 seconds
Side plank (stacked feet)	15 seconds each side

BRACKET 3: Average

Plank	30 seconds
Raise left arm and right leg	15 seconds
Raise right arm and left leg	15 seconds
Side plank with hip raise (stacked feet)	10 reps each side

BRACKET 4: Advanced

Plank	30 seconds
Raise left arm and right leg and crunch both in before returning	5 reps
Raise right arm and left leg and crunch both in before returning	5 reps
Side plank (stacked feet)	20 seconds each side
Side plank with reach under rotations	10 reps each side
Side plank with top leg drive (knee toward chest)	5 reps each side

BRACKET 5: Superior

Plank	45 seconds
Raise left arm and right leg and crunch both in before returning	5 reps
Raise right arm and left leg and crunch both in before returning	5 reps
Side plank (stacked feet)	30 seconds each side
Side plank with hip raise then reach under rotation	5 reps each side
Side plank with leg drive and leg raise	5 reps each side

BRACKET 6: Elite

Plank	60 seconds
Raise left arm and right leg and crunch both in before returning	10 reps
Raise right arm and left leg and crunch both in before returning	10 reps
Side plank with hip raise and reach under rotation	10 reps each side
Side plank with double leg drive (staggered /split feet)	5 reps each side

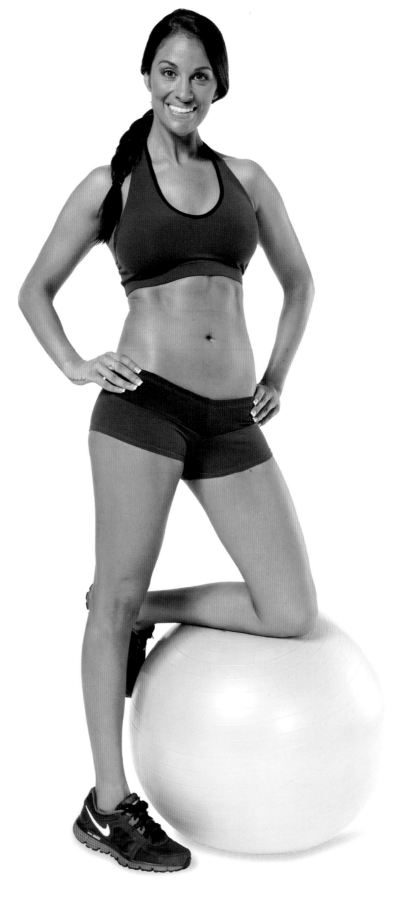

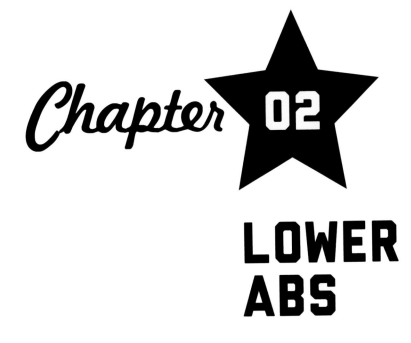

Chapter 02

LOWER ABS

WHERE DO MOST PEOPLE STORE FAT? THE MIDSECTION. ALSO REFERRED TO AS THE LOWER ABS. YOUR LOWER ABS ARE LOCATED BELOW YOUR BELT AND BELLY BUTTON AND ARE A PART OF THE RECTUS ABDOMINIS MUSCLE. BUT, IF YOU THINK THAT DOING A LOT OF LOWER ABS WORK WILL RESULT IN LOSING FAT IN THAT SPECIFIC AREA. YOU'RE WRONG.

Spot training to remove fat in this problematic area isn't going to work, but it can still generate results—especially when you're trying to strengthen your core. And, when it comes to your overall core strength, the lower abs are the weakest and most underused muscles you've got. Targeting your lower abs will result in working your hip flexors—it's a by-product of the movements that you have to do in order to effectively move said muscles. If you're a sprinter, or in a sport that requires bursts of speed, this is a great benefit. If you're not an athlete, you're going to find this

section of the book particularly challenging. Why? Because your lower abs are less developed and, as a result, you're going to have a very hard time harnessing the power within them to properly engage them throughout your sets. Our advice is to start with your lower abs exercises so you don't tire them out before even getting to them and to always begin with the easiest movements, focusing more on the form of each exercise and making sure your abs are engaged, rather than performing a multitude of reps or adding weight.

1. PELVIC TILT

Brace yourself! This is the foundation of your abdominal strength for movement, absorbing impact, sports performance, unanticipated movements, and more. In combination with engaging your glutes, bracing your abs is the "power-on switch" you need for your Core Fitness Solution.

BEGINNER

Although some trainers may suggest that you rest your calf muscles on a bench to minimize the use of your legs in this movement, we feel more focus needs to be put on specifically maintaining a neutral alignment of your lower back against the floor by:

1) bracing your lower abs and pulling your hips up toward your ribs, resulting in your back pressing against the floor.

2) squeezing your glutes, to assist your abdominal muscles, without lifting them off of the floor.

(Holding the tilt for 2 seconds and relaxing is considered one repetition.)

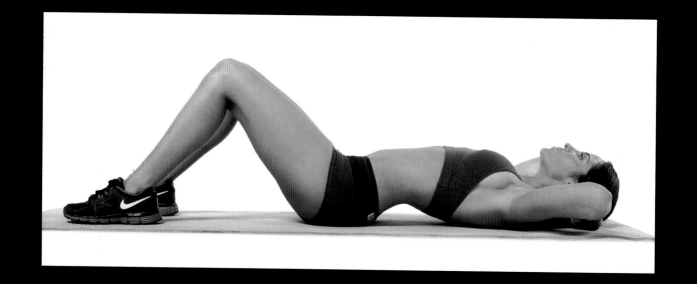

START Lie on your back with your feet flat on the floor, retaining the slight arch that naturally occurs in your lower back when lying on a flat surface.

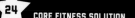

ADVANCED

Stand in a shallow squat/hip hinge and hold the pelvic tilt position for 90 seconds.

Brace your lower abs so your naval is slightly drawn inward toward your spine, while simultaneously tilting your pelvis. Additionally, squeeze your glutes, which should result in your spine being flat on the floor (without lifting your butt off of the ground). Practice until you can hold the position at peak contraction for 60 seconds.

SUCK IT IN

Another great foundational abdominal exercise is the Draw-In Maneuver, a.k.a. Abdominal Hollowing. This is very similar to the vacuum pose in bodybuilding, and it is also used in yoga and Pilates practices. Begin by lying on the floor and progress to a standing position for additional difficulty. Pulling your belly button in toward your spine, and holding, works your transverse abdominus and multifidus muscles. Practice without holding your breath. Although we recommend that you include this great move in your program, we suggest that your primary fundamental position to support movement should be bracing for movement exercises and drawing-in for stability exercises.

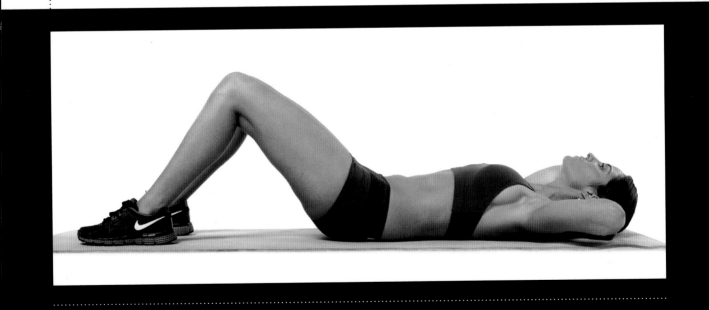

2. AB CRUNCH WITH VERTICAL LEGS

Because there is so little movement in this exercise, most people might think that it ranks as one of the easiest. But, if you're finding it to be easy, you're doing it wrong. Focus on the motion with an emphasis on your lower abs and you'll feel every inch of this move in your core.

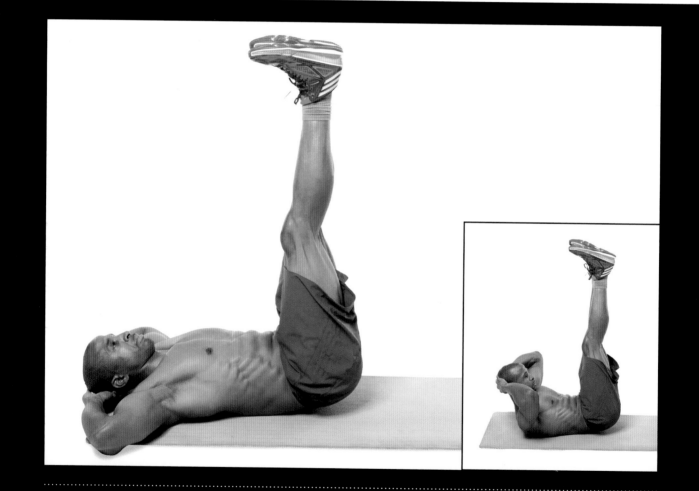

START Lie flat on your back with your hands cradling your skull. Bring your legs up so the soles of your feet are parallel to the ceiling. Keep your legs straight and heels together.

BEGINNER

Make this move easier by keeping a 90-degree bend in your knees throughout each rep. At the start, your calf muscles are parallel with the floor; as you bring your legs lower, do not let your feet touch the ground.

ADVANCED

Kick the intensity of this move up a notch by adding an upward thrust to the end of each rep so your hip and upper buttocks leave the floor (see inset).This is a very small movement of only a couple of inches. Don't use momentum. Harness the power of your lower abs to thrust your legs upward.

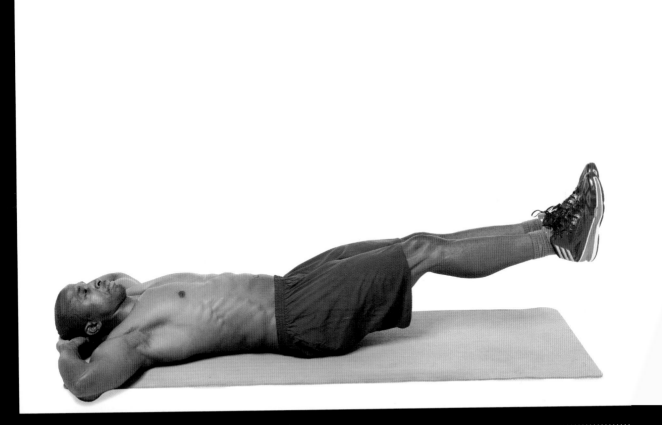

ACTION Slowly lower your legs until your heels are a few inches off the ground. Do not let your feet drop while you're doing this movement. From there, raise your legs back up to the starting position while crunching forward with your upper body, being sure not to pull with your hands. That is one rep. Remember to keep your legs straight and together throughout the entire movement. Do not swing

3. U-BOAT

Perhaps one of the most complex moves you'll ever do, this exercise might turn you off at first because of its complicated U-like movement. Mastering it, however, will yield great results. Our advice: Even if you're an advanced trainer, start with the beginner's tip to prepare yourself.

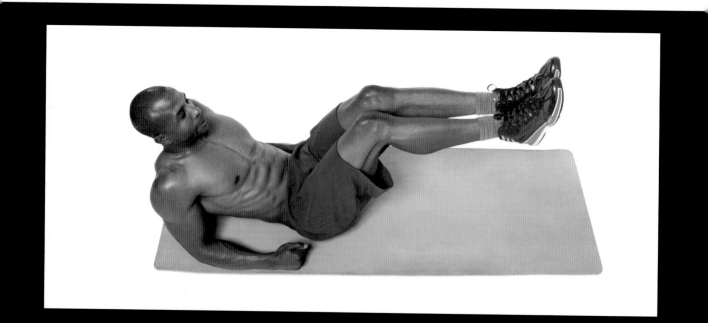

START Lie flat so your butt, fists and forearms (elbows to fists) are the only parts of your anatomy touching the floor. Keeping your spine straight, make a 45-degree angle with the floor.

ACTION Keeping your knees together and bent, use the power in your lower abs to bring your legs up so your shins are parallel to the ceiling. From there, move your legs to the left so they make a 45-degree angle to the ground. Then, move your legs to the right while straightening your knees slightly, which will create a U-like motion as you bring your legs back up on the opposite side.

BEGINNER

Make this move a little easier by lying flat on the floor and keeping your arms at your sides. This will ensure that you still put the focus on your lower abs, but no longer have to balance your body as described below.

ADVANCED

If you've mastered this movement and want to add even more intensity, we recommend holding a V-sit so your body is no longer being balanced by your forearms. Keep your hands straight up, pointing toward the ceiling, throughout each rep.

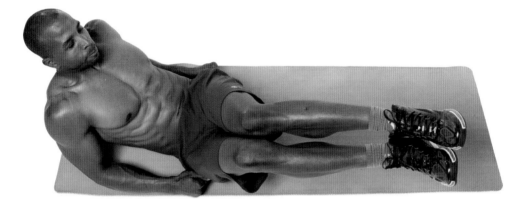

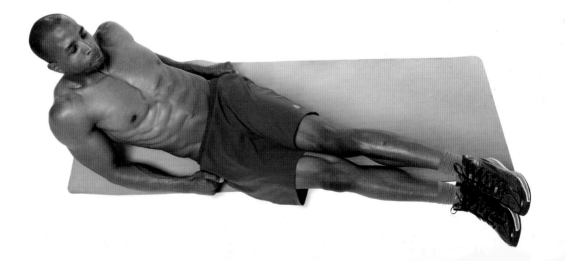

HINT

The motion that you're doing in this exercise isn't simple. In fact, without practice, it is very easy to never fully realize the true potential of this movement. Our advice is to do it with your eyes closed, visualizing the movement of your legs making an imaginary "U" in the air for each rep. Your mind will guide your muscles to make the proper contractions and you won't be distracted with how you look or what else is in the room.

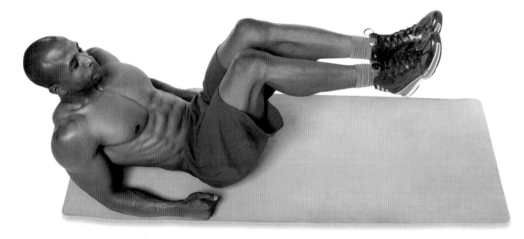

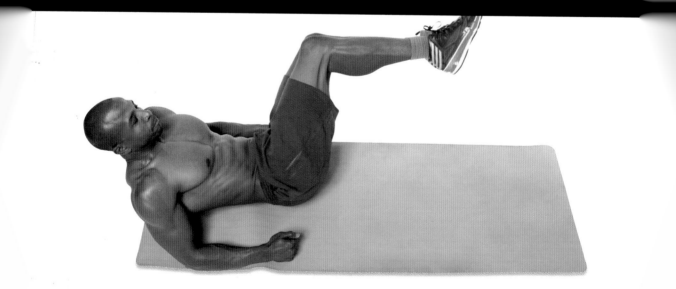

FOCUS

Because there's a lot to keep in mind when you're doing the U-Boat, we won't add in anything more to retain through the movement. Instead, prioritize. Sure, there's a lot to do, but do things in a progression. New to the move? Keep your arms flat on the ground. Not getting the move? Try breaking it into sections. Above all, however, focus on keeping your ankles and knees together throughout the reps.

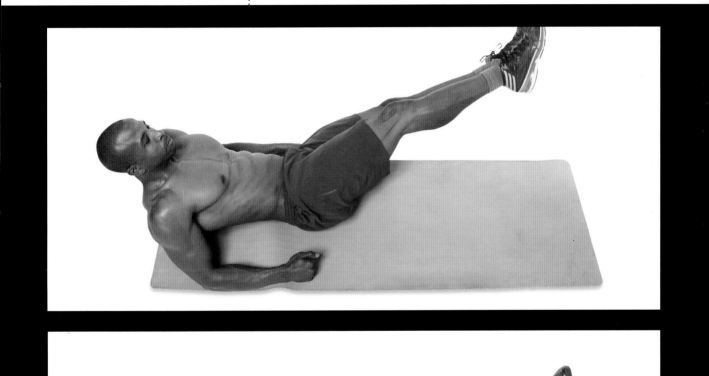

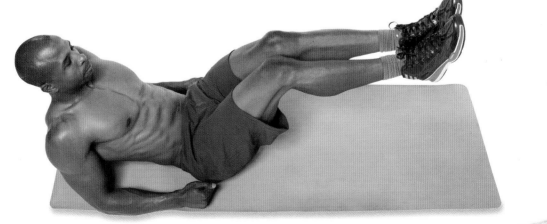

4. FIGURE FOUR LEG RAISE AND CRUNCH

Named for the shape it puts your legs in, the figure four leg raise will have you wanting to cheat with your oblique muscles to perform each rep. Stick with steady movements through each rep for best results. Because it provides a hip flexor stretch, this move is especially crucial for athletes in high-impact sports with lots of running, such as football.

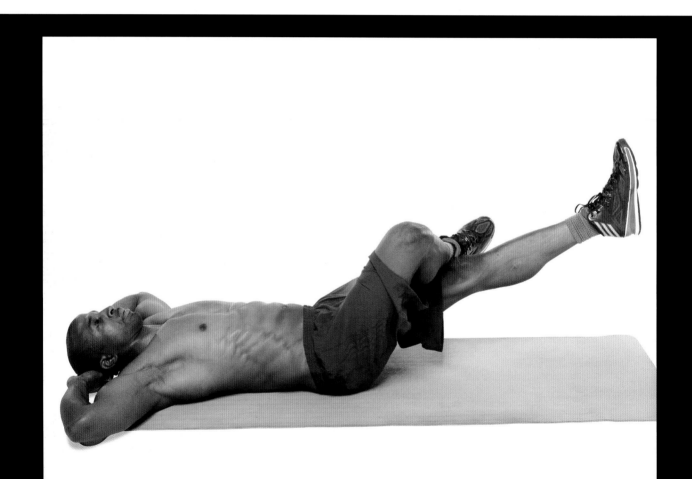

START Lie flat on your back in a typical crunch position with your hands behind your head. Stretch your left leg straight out, creating

BEGINNER

If you're finding this move too difficult, don't put one ankle on the opposite knee. Instead, just raise one leg at a time, leaving the opposite foot flat on the ground.

ADVANCED

Make this move more difficult by adding ankle weights for more resistance.

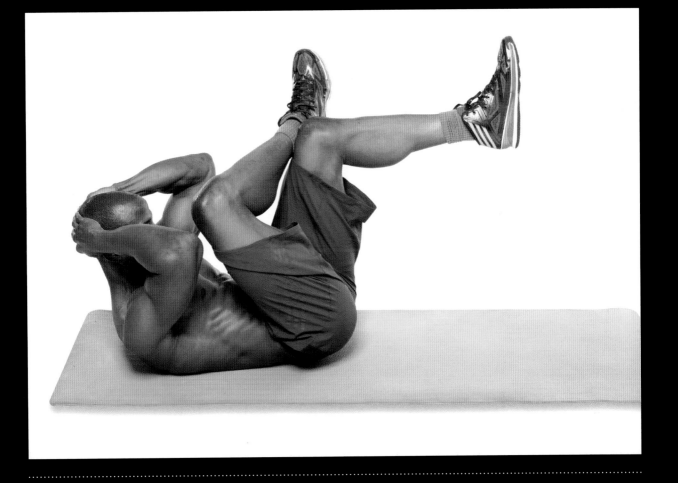

ACTION Keeping your ankle on your knee, bring your legs forward while crunching your upper body upward. Do not swing your legs to complete the move.

5. CAPTAIN'S CHAIR LEG LIFT

This is one of the few exercises in this book that requires gym equipment. You'll need access to a captain's chair or parallel bars in order to complete your sets. We included this exercise because of how effective it is in targeting the lower abs, but it is also one of the easiest exercises to lose your focus and not actually work the intended muscles. Take this exercise on once you've reached a higher comfort level with your training.

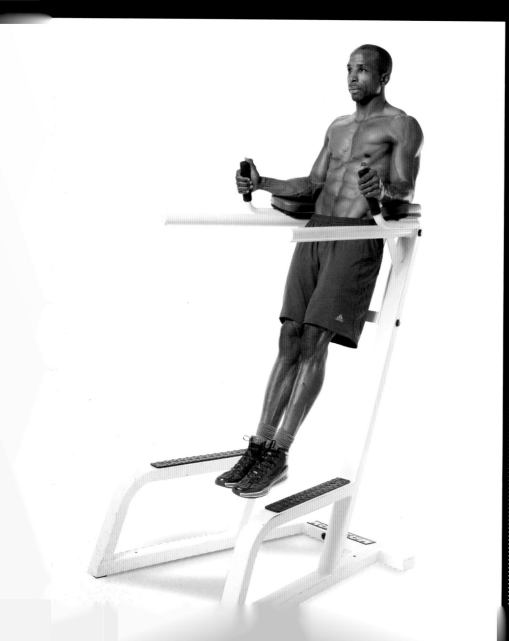

START

Position yourself in a captain's chair with your forearms flat against the cushions and your hands firmly gripping the handles. Tilt your pelvis and keep your feet slightly in front of your hips for proper lower abdominal engagement.

BEGINNER

Alternate your legs during this movement to make it easier, but do not create an angle in your crunching motion that favors either side.

ADVANCED

Squeeze a dumbbell or medicine ball between your legs to add more intensity to this move. For even more intensity, kick your legs out during each rep so you create an L shape (or a V shape while lifting your tailbone away from the chair).

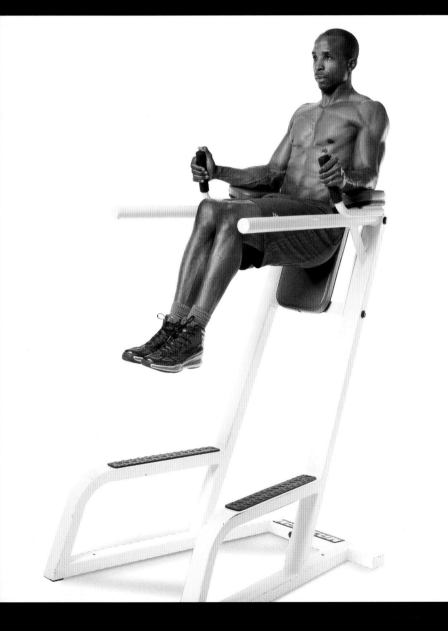

ACTION

Crunch your legs up toward your torso so your hamstrings are parallel to the floor and your knees create a 90-degree angle or higher in your legs. Look straight ahead throughout the movement. Slowly return your legs to the starting position but do not let your feet go under your hips. Always lift from the bottom with the power of your lower abs.

6. HANGING LEG RAISE

You'll need a chin-up bar for this move and a great deal of patience. Although this exercise can be done quickly, the best results come from a very methodical upward and downward motion with a focus on your lower abs throughout. Because you're also holding your entire weight on the bar, consider this a test of your upper body, grip, and arm strength all in one. Enjoy.

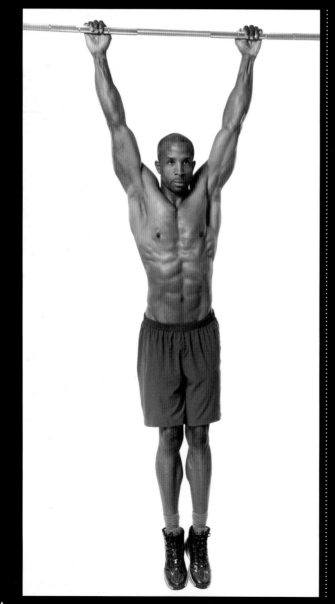

START

Hold your weight on a chin-up bar with your arms shoulder-width apart. Let your legs dangle directly downward so the soles of your feet are parallel to the floor.

BEGINNER

Make this move easier
by alternating your legs.
Remember to keep your body
straight throughout the set and
resist the urge to twist to either
side to complete your reps.

ADVANCED

Add ankle weights to
increase the intensity of
this move.

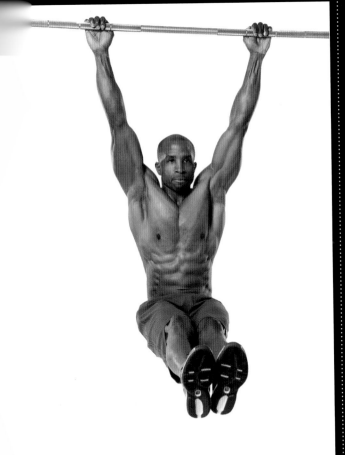

ACTION

Crunch your legs up toward your
torso so your hamstrings are
parallel to the floor. Do not bring
your knees past your hips and
look straight ahead throughout
the movement. Slowly return
your legs to the starting position
without using momentum.

7. FLUTTER KICKS

Flutter kicks may sound a little too light to be in a challenging fitness book like this, but performing flutter kicks from the safety of the floor is a great way to harness the power of your lower abs. If you're a boxer or competitive dancer, focus on the speed of your kicks to help with your footwork.

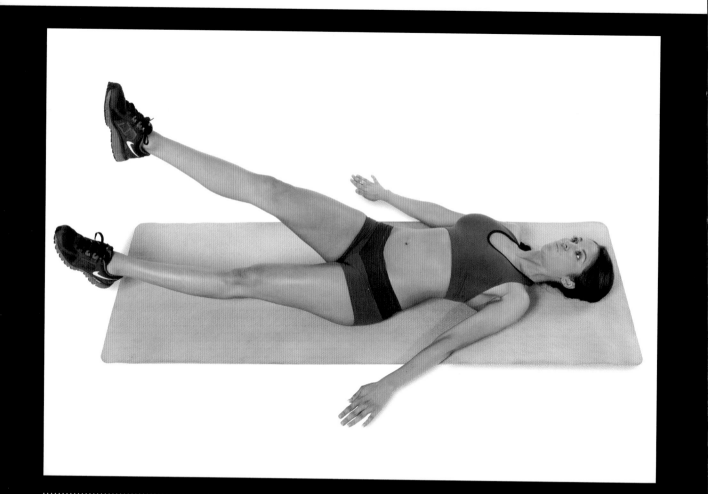

START Lie flat on your back with your arms at your sides for balance. Lift your legs off the ground in an open-scissor position, making a 45-degree angle with the floor, and keep them aligned.

BEGINNER

Make this move a little easier by starting with your legs at an angle closer to the floor, but do not allow them to make contact with the ground.

ADVANCED

Make this move harder by moving your legs up and down methodically through each rep. Focus on keeping your legs between a 45- and 90-degree angle to the floor, but remember to kick each leg up and down for each rep. You can also scissor kick your legs (kicking left to right) open and closed or across each other for further intensity.

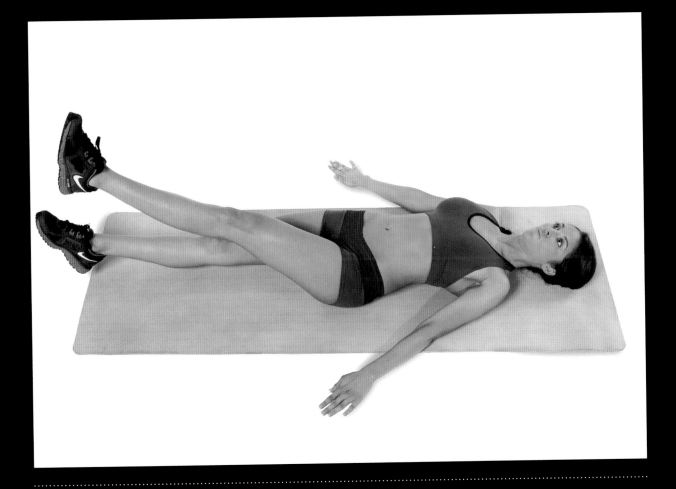

ACTION Keeping your back, shoulders, and arms flat on the floor throughout each rep, kick your legs in alternating rhythm to mimic scissors. Each leg goes up and down to perform one rep. Do not bend your knees at all throughout the set.

8. VERTICAL LEG CRUNCH

While this exercise may look like a simple move, you will be prone to injury if you do not stay true to form. Make sure you don't bounce on your tailbone throughout your reps.

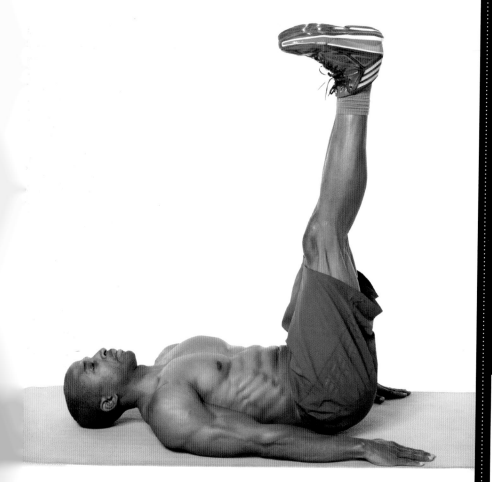

START
Lie flat on the floor with your arms at your sides and your legs up (soles parallel to the ceiling). For balance, open your hands and keep them, palms down, at your sides.

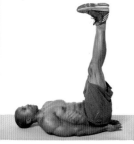

BEGINNER

Put your hands under the small of your back to make this move a little easier and to offer more stability through each rep (see inset).

ADVANCED

Kick up the intensity of this move by adding weight. You can cradle a dumbbell between your feet or use resistance bands.

ACTION

Thrust your feet up toward the ceiling. Your lower back and buttocks should only move a few inches off the ground. Focus the contraction on your upper abs. Keep a very meticulous pace through your reps, being careful not to bounce your lower back on the floor.

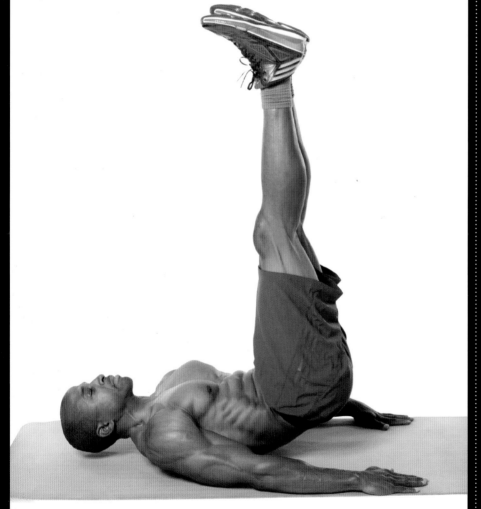

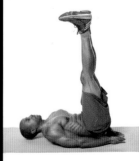

9. BENCH LEG RAISE

You can do this move on just about any flat, cushioned surface, but we recommend a weight bench. If you're adding intensity to this move by using a dumbbell, make sure it is secure between your feet at all times.

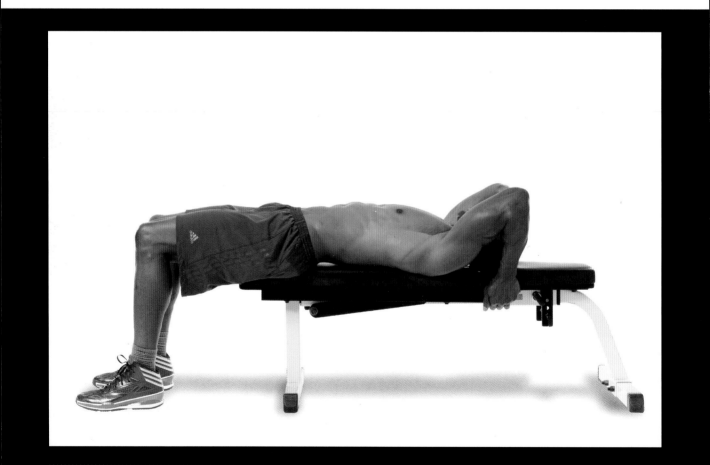

START Lie on a bench with your back flat and your butt on the edge of the bench, but still supported. Keep your arms at your sides or reach back and hold the top of the bench for balance. Your feet are flat on the floor and your knees bent at 90 degrees.

BEGINNER

Make this move easier by bending your knees during the crunching motion so your toes are pointing up and your shins are parallel to the ceiling.

ADVANCED

There are several ways to make this move more intense. Our favorite is pausing and holding a contraction in three spots while bringing your legs down to the starting position. You can also add ankle weights or hold a dumbbell or medicine ball between your feet.

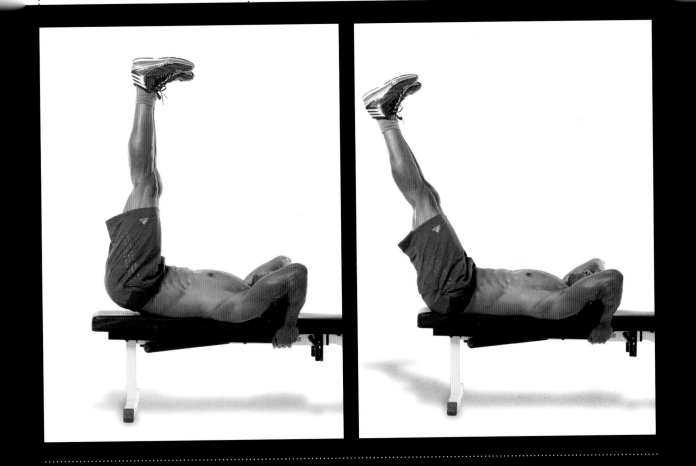

ACTION Kick out your legs so you make a straight line with your body; point your toes toward the ceiling. Crunch your legs up toward your torso. Keep your legs straight throughout the movement and stop when the soles of your feet are parallel to the ceiling. Do not arch your back or pull with

HINT

You're going to really have to fight every impulse you've got to retain proper form and contraction to do this move properly. Most people will pull and use their arms, upper back, and shoulders to perform the rep. Don't. Instead, use the power of your abs throughout, making sure to perform every contraction with meticulous attention to detail.

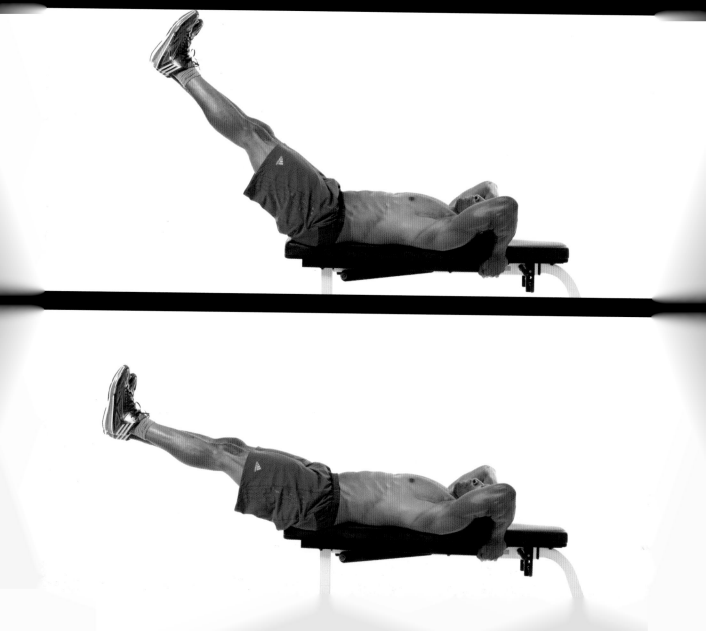

10. RECLINING LEG CIRCLES

The circular motion in each rep will harness all of your core, while the lowering and raising of your legs will specifically target your lower abs. The key to this movement is to make sure that your leg circles are conducted in an even, methodical manner. Don't rush or make fast circles to make the reps easier.

BEGINNER

Make this move a little easier by starting with your legs straight up, so the soles of your feet are parallel to the ceiling. Remember not to let momentum aid in your movement and to keep your upper body flat on the ground.

ADVANCED

Perform this movement in exactly the same manner listed above, but start each rep with your heels just a few inches off the ground and return them to that same spot at the conclusion of each rep.

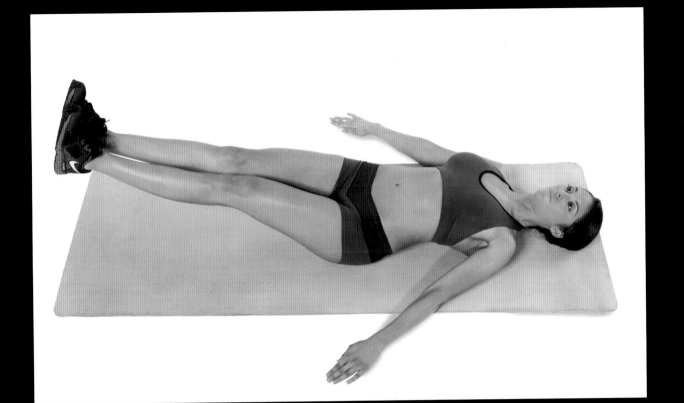

START Lie flat on your back with your arms at your sides for balance. Lift your legs off the ground, making a 45-degree angle with the floor.

ACTION Keeping your legs and feet together, rotate your legs in a circular motion while lowering them toward the ground, stopping a few inches, before making contact. Remember to keep your back, shoulders, and arms flat on the floor throughout each rep.

11. HOVER

This one may look easy, but appearances are definitely deceiving when it comes to this lower abs assault. Much of this exercise is based on your being honest with your movement. Don't rock on your heels to create momentum or rely on your spine or upper body to move your torso forward to mimic the intended motion of this move. Instead, be extra mindful of bracing your lower abs, forcing them to do all the work. Once you have that mind-muscle connection, you'll be feeling your lower abs as never before.

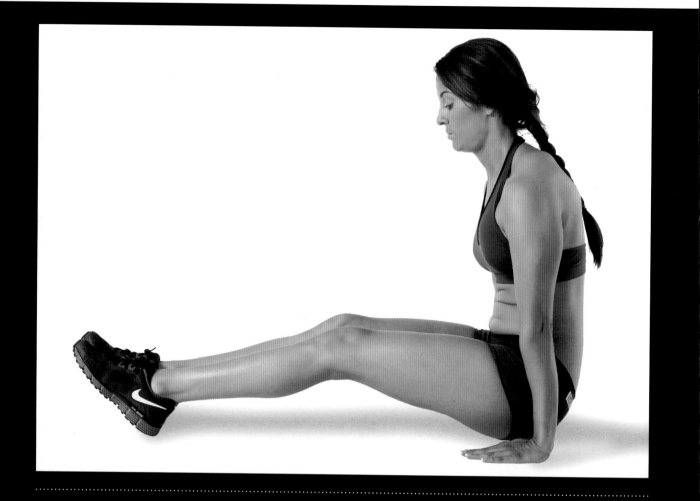

START Sit on the floor with your legs pointing straight ahead of you and your toes pointing at the ceiling. Put your hands by your hips and place them flat on the floor with your palms down.

BEGINNER

You can alternate your leg placement during this movement to make it easier. Simply leave one leg flat on the floor while the other is balanced on your heel.

ADVANCED

Adding a weight plate to your lap will create more tension in this exercise. Also, instead of returning to the starting position (where your legs are flat on the floor), for added intensity, try to stay off the ground for as many reps as possible.

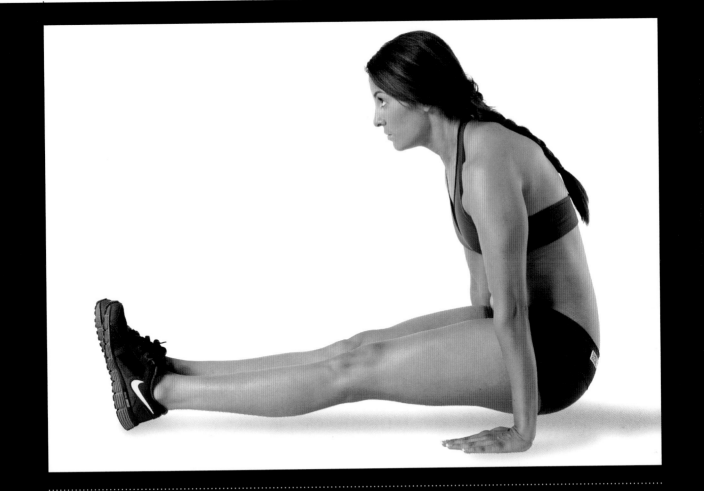

ACTION Push down with your hands to raise your butt off the floor so only your hands and heels are touching the ground. With a slight bend in your knees, contract your abs inward and use the power of your lower abs to push your hips backward so they move to just behind your shoulders, making your spine angled at about 80 degrees.

12. TOES TO BAR HANGING LEG RAISE

This is a bonus exercise for extremely advanced trainers. One of our favorite exercises in this book is the hanging leg raise. If done correctly, it can create overall core strength and definition that few exercises can compare with. That's why we covered it earlier in this chapter. The reason we're setting this variation apart from the earlier movement is when it comes to overall core strength and total body power, it's simply one of the best challenges possible for advanced trainers and elite athletes. If you can do this one, you need to let us know and show it off!

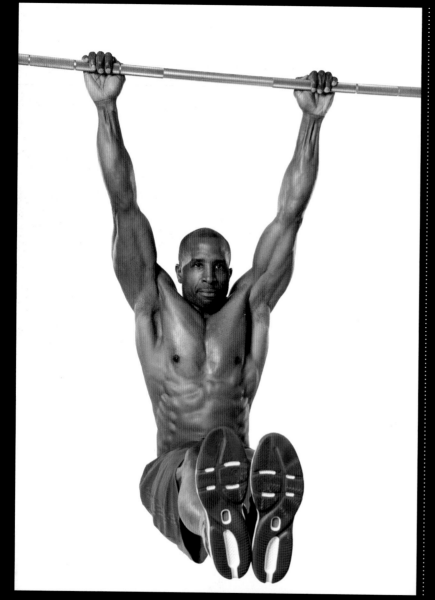

START
As with the regular hanging leg raise, hold your weight on a chin-up bar with your arms shoulder-width apart. Let your legs dangle directly downward so the soles of your feet are parallel to the floor.

There are no beginner or advanced tips for this move. This is an elite movement. Just remember: You should be able to handle dozens of regular hanging leg raises before entertaining the thought of adding this move to your repertoire.

ACTION

Crunch your legs up toward your torso so your front thighs reach your chest and your toes reach the bar that you're holding your weight on. Slowly return your legs to the starting position without using momentum.

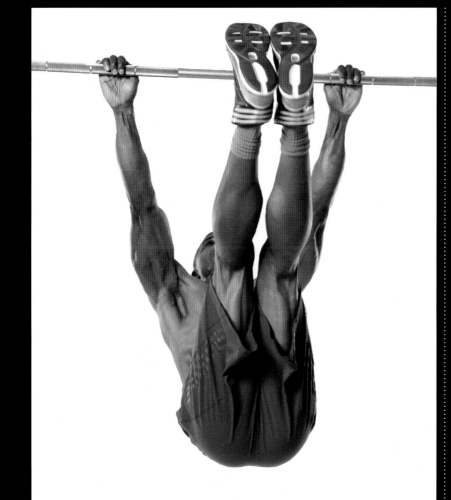

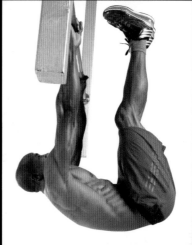

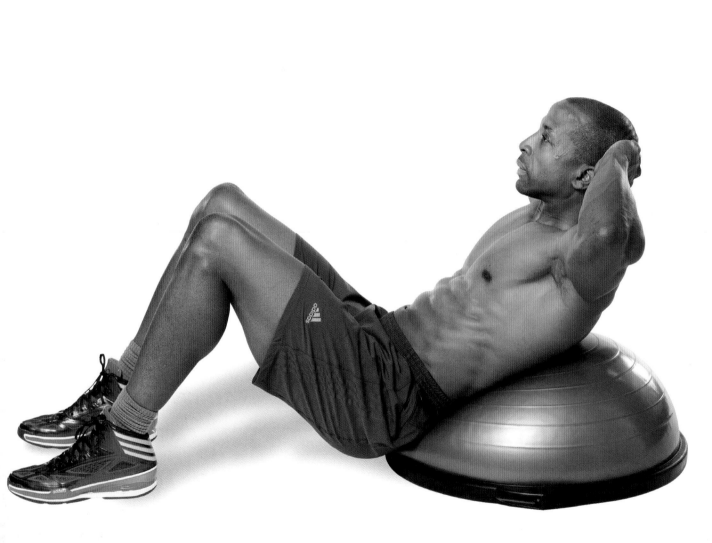

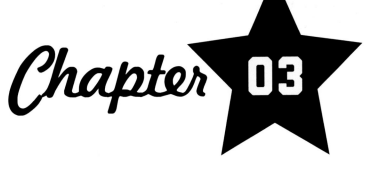

Chapter 03

UPPER ABS

PUT YOUR HANDS JUST UNDER YOUR PECS. FEEL THAT? THESE ARE YOU UPPER ABS.

The muscle you're feeling is the upper part of the rectus abdominis, which is a long muscle that extends to the bottom of your core and to the left and right, where it meets the obliques on either side. If you tense your core, you'll probably feel some flexing under your hands in this area and quite possibly nowhere else. Why? Chances are you're strongest in your upper abs area. When you move your torso forward, down toward your legs or even brace for any movement, you're using your upper abs. Because you're probably already strongest in this area, you may find that you seem more advanced in this section of the book. And you're probably right. But don't let your stats from this chapter be a benchmark for the others.

1. CRUNCH AND REACH

When people see the word *crunch*, many immediately think they have to bring their entire spine off the ground and swing their weight around wildly. A proper crunch (with reach or not) is a very meticulous move with subtle motions. All you need is a flat surface and a serious emphasis on the form (see below).

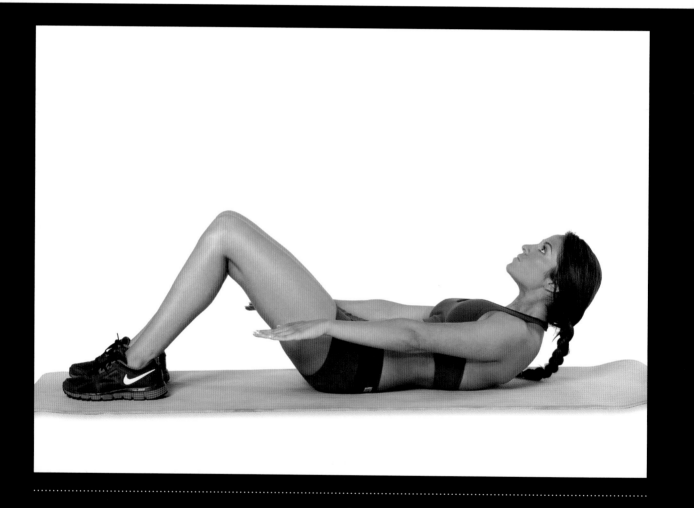

START Lie face up on the floor with your spine straight, legs bent at the knee and arms pointing toward the far wall. Do not tuck your chin against your chest; keep your neck in line with your spine.

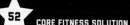

BEGINNER

Put your hands behind your head, cradling your skull. Crunch forward, but do not pull with your arms or hands.

ADVANCED

Lift one leg off the ground, alternating with each repetition, so that your calf is parallel to the floor (see photo below).

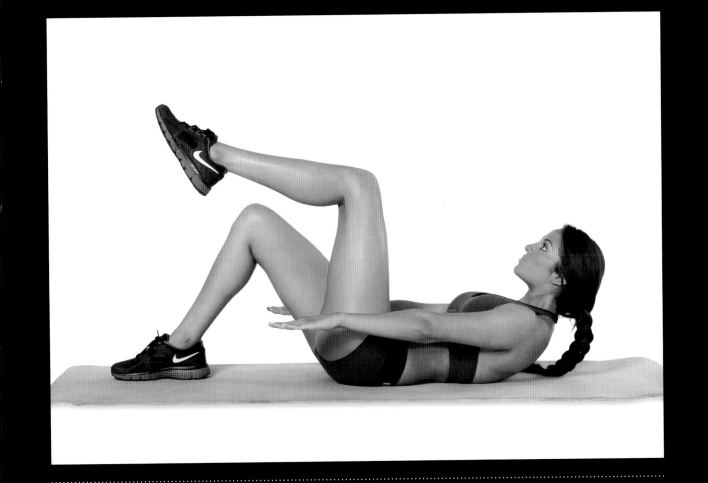

ACTION Crunch your upper torso up and forward. The movement brings your shoulders a few inches off the ground while your lower back and feet remain flat. Keep your arms pointing at the far wall as you move up and down in the crunching motion.

2. DEAD BUG

This move may have an odd name and funny starting position, but it's seriously challenging with definite core-building benefits. All you need is a flat surface and a great deal of core stability to get through your reps.

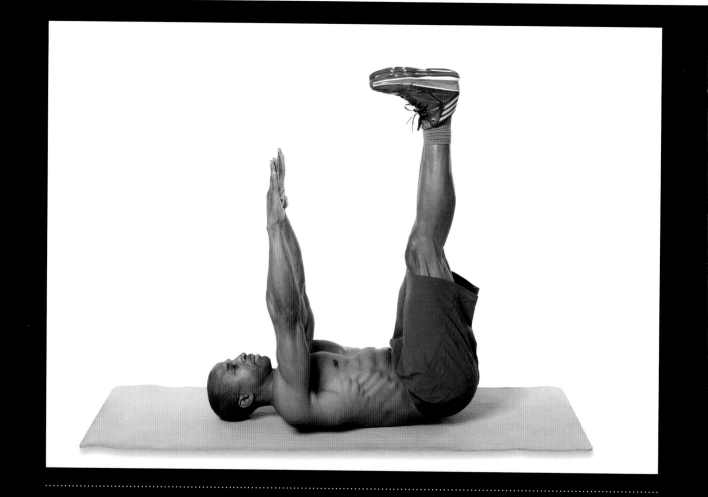

START Lie on the floor with your spine flat and your legs up so the soles of your feet are pointing to the ceiling. Point your arms straight up.

BEGINNER

To make this move easier, lie flat between each repetition so you are not in constant contraction.

ADVANCED

Hold this move for a count of two on each repetition. You can also bend your knees at a 90-degree angle.

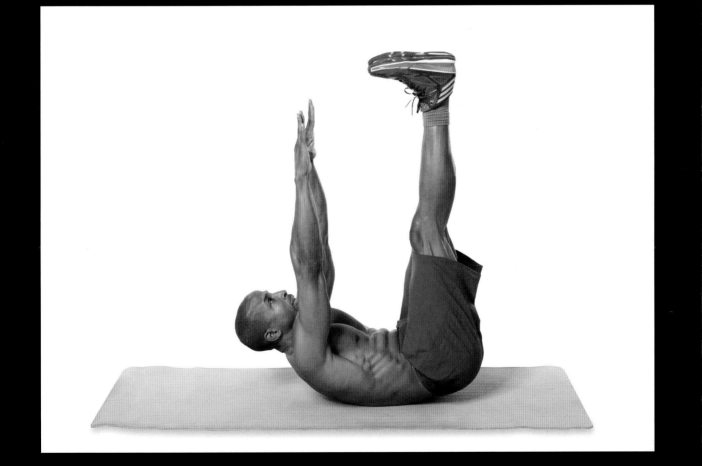

ACTION Slowly crunch your upper body forward while maintaining your leg position

3. STABILITY BALL CRUNCH

Stability balls are a great tool for building core strength, but they've also become a gym gimmick that gets added to almost any exercise you can imagine. The result: injuries. We advise using the stability ball on selected crunches because your feet remain flat on the floor to retain balance. If, however, you're not sure of your balance, the Bosu ball is the perfect solution.

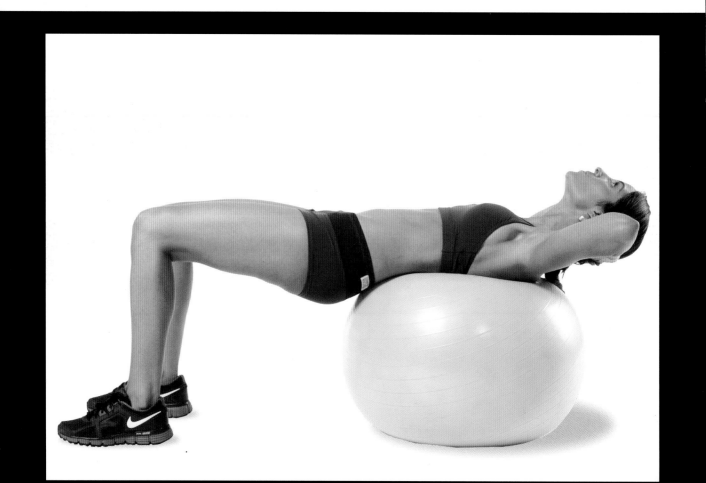

START Lie on a balance ball so your spine is fully cradled. Be careful with your positioning

BEGINNER
If balancing on the stability ball is too difficult, lie on a Bosu ball (round side up) to minimize the chance of rolling off.

ADVANCED
If you've mastered balancing on the ball, point your arms straight up at the ceiling through each rep.

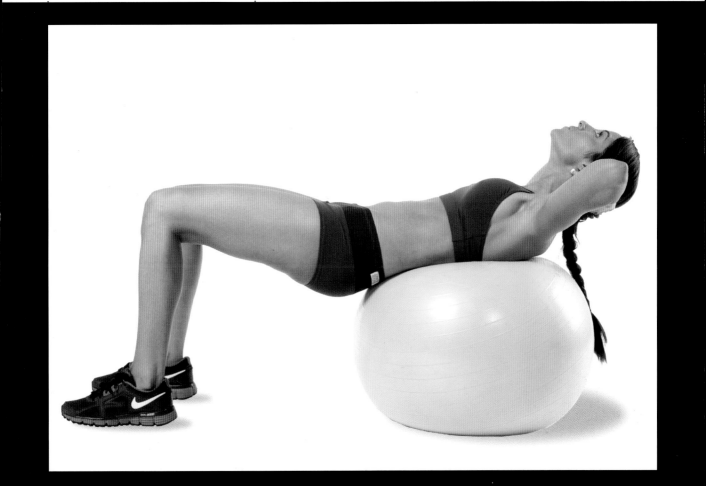

ACTION Crunch your upper torso forward, while maintaining your feet flat on the floor. Do not pull with your arms or hands.

4. DOUBLE CRUNCH

The double crunch may be the quintessential abdominal movement. It targets the upper abs while also harnessing other areas of your core. All you need is a flat surface.

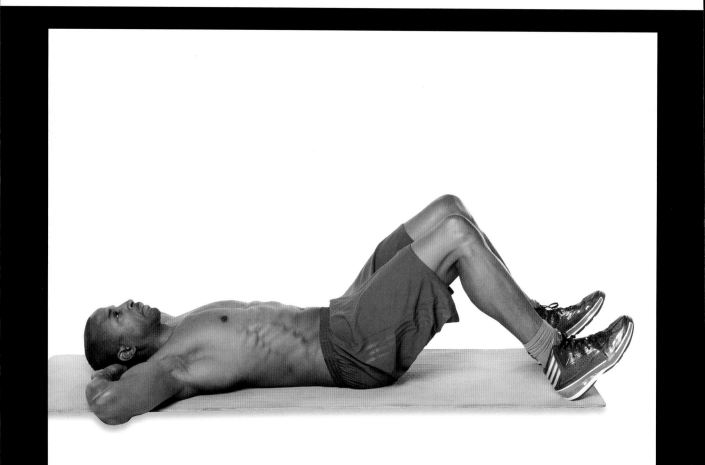

START Lie on the floor so your back and heels are on the ground with your legs bent at the knee. Cradle your skull with your hands behind

BEGINNER

To make this move a little easier, start with your calves resting on a bench for each repetition.

ADVANCED

Hold the contraction for two counts to get more out of this exercise.

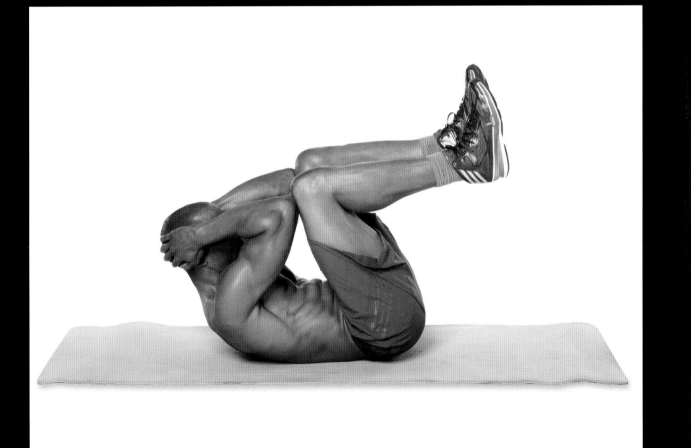

ACTION Crunch your upper torso forward while simultaneously bringing your knees toward your chest. Try to get your elbows to touch your knees to complete a rep. Do not jerk forward with your hands. Slowly lower your upper body and legs back to the starting position.

5. BOSU BALL CRUNCH

The Bosu ball might be the lesser-known cousin of the stability ball, but it should never be overlooked. In fact, the Bosu is a much better tool for most people because it eliminates many slip-and-fall injuries that can occur when doing this type of training. Try the standard crunch on the Bosu for more range of motion and see the results.

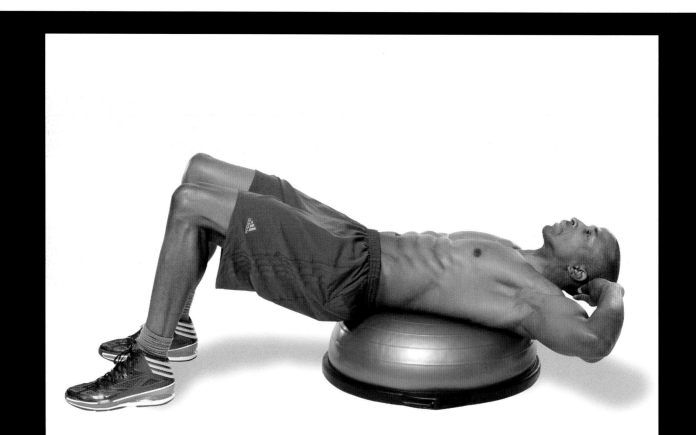

START Lie on the Bosu ball in a standard crunch

HINT

"Slipping of the Bosu ball" is something that's become a thing of comedy in a lot of gyms. Give it a good wipe before getting on it and make sure that your butt isn't on the floor. If you're finding that difficult, put a towel under your workout area to provide more friction while you're sitting and crunching.

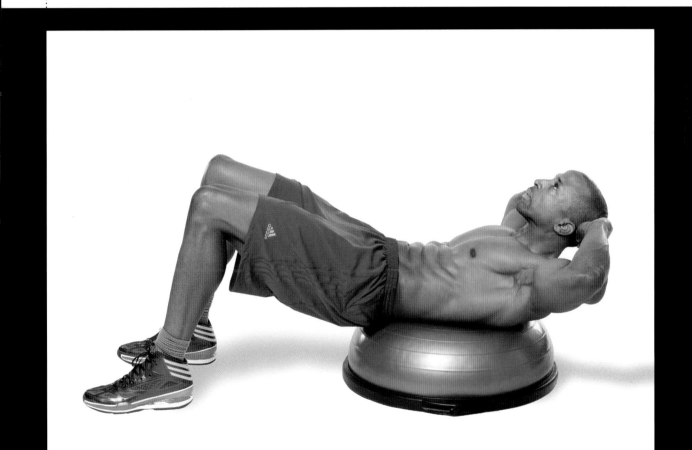

ACTION Crunch your upper body forward, but do

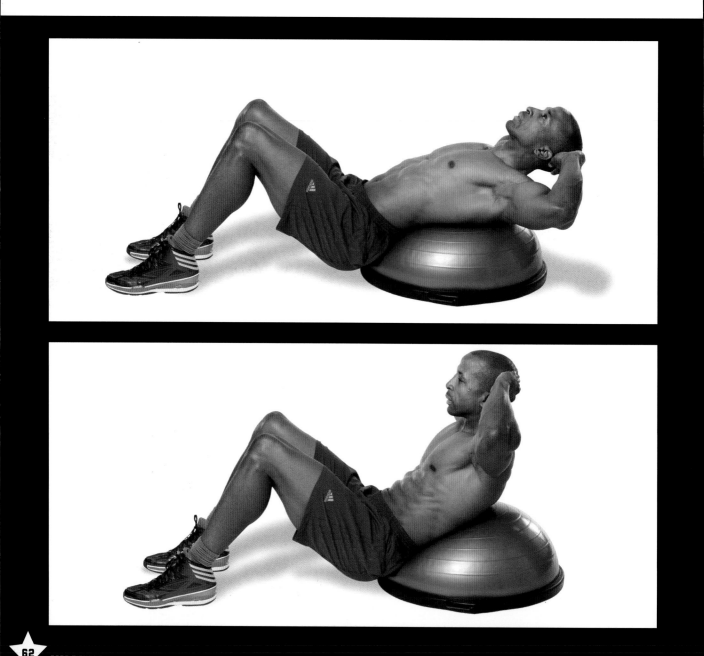

BEGINNER

Lower your butt closer to the rim of the Bosu ball (just above the floor) to make this crunch easier.

ADVANCED

Cradle a dumbbell behind your head and perform the crunch as described above to add intensity to this exercise.

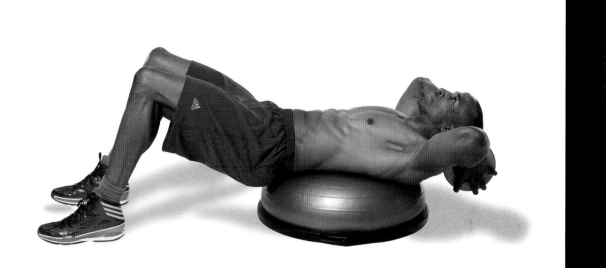

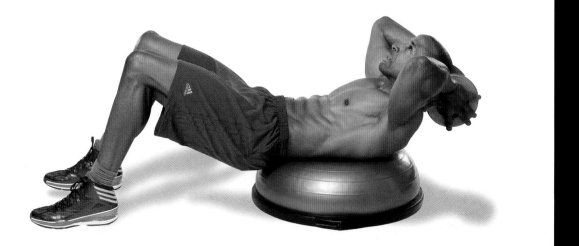

6. LEG CLIMB

Often overlooked by most trainers, this movement is great for your upper abs because it can be accomplished at any fitness level and only requires a flat surface.

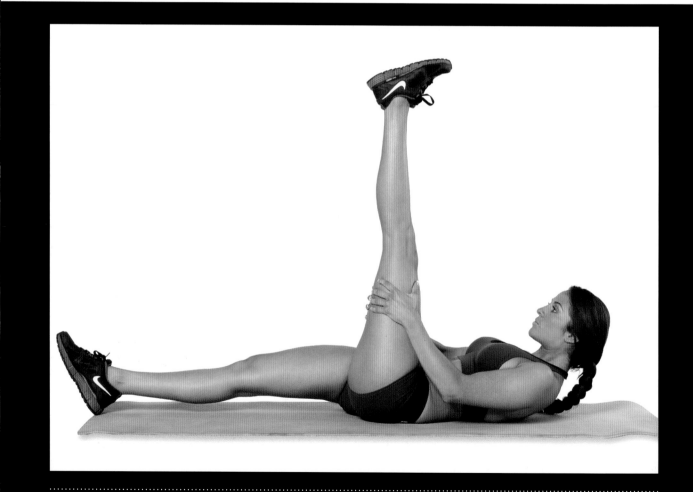

START Lie flat on the floor with your right leg stretched out and your left leg up so the sole of your foot is parallel to the ceiling.

BEGINNER

Instead of reaching up your leg four times, gradually move your grip toward your ankle only twice per rep (because you have only two reaches, it's not expected that you will reach your ankle).

ADVANCED

Add intensity to this move by upping your reaches from four to six on each leg.

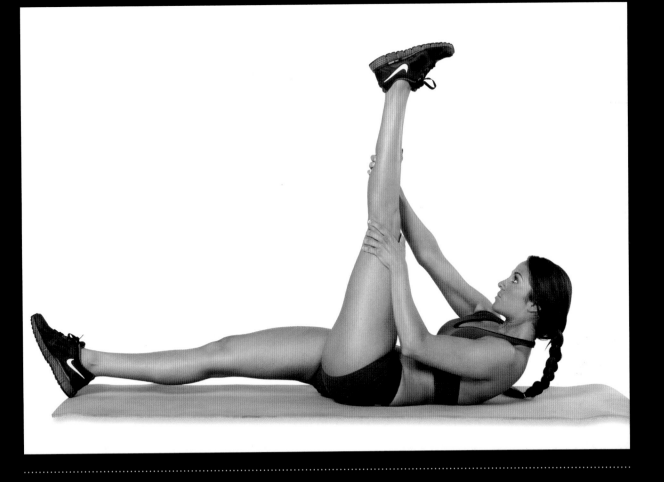

ACTION Reach your arms forward so your hands cradle the back of your left thigh. Gradually move your hands up your leg in four reaches so your hands are as close to your ankle as possible. Repeat with your other leg.

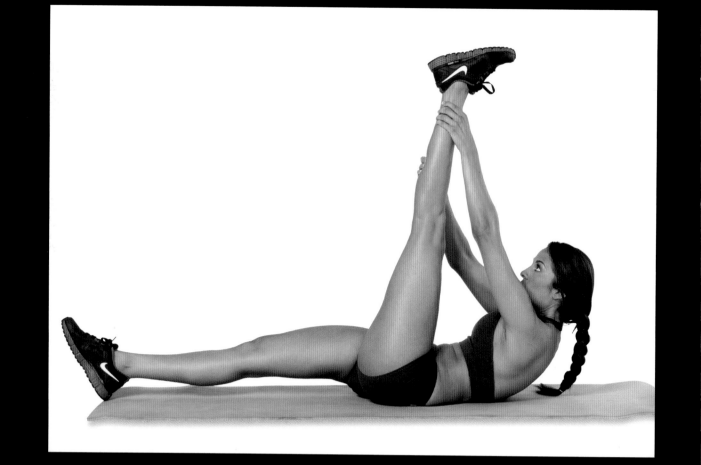

7. WEIGHTED CRUNCH

Just because you've mastered the crunch doesn't mean you get to cut it from your repertoire. Add some weight to the movement and you'll feel like a novice all over again. All you need is a weight plate (or dumbbell) and a flat surface.

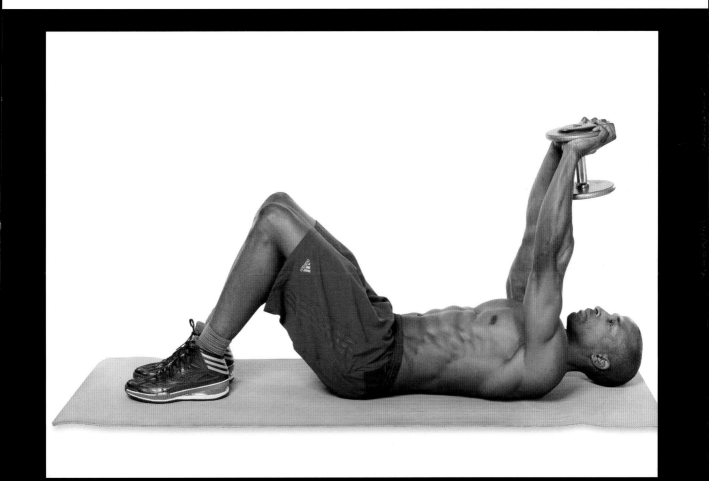

START Lie flat on the floor with your knees bent while hugging a weight plate to your chest or holding a weight plate or dumbbell

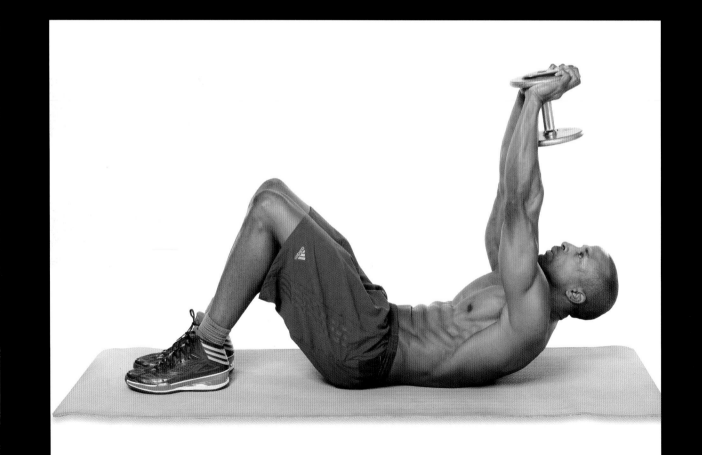

BEGINNER

If the additional weight is too much, perform the movement without any weight while cradling your skull with your hands behind your head.

ADVANCED

Perform each rep in the same manner as described in basic move, but bring one leg up on each rep. Alternate your legs and keep them straight, with your calves parallel to the ground. Do not angle your legs inward (see photo below).

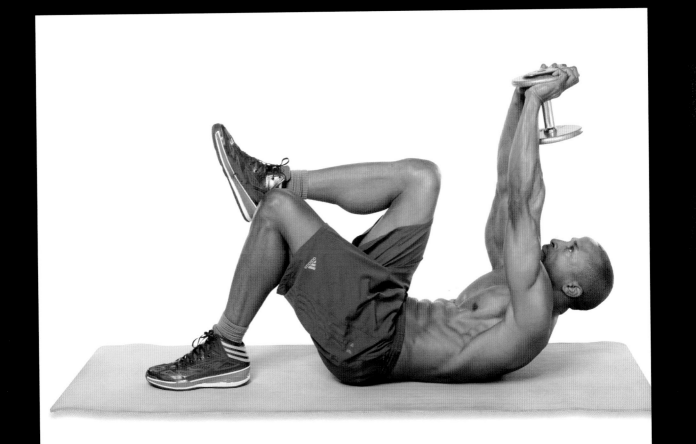

8. KNEELING RESISTANCE BAND CRUNCH

You know those resistance bands that you thought were pool toys or random pieces of plastic at the gym? They're great tools for adding resistance to any movement. Follow the color guide to select the right one for you: Yellow is easiest, red is a bit harder, green is harder, and blue is most advanced.

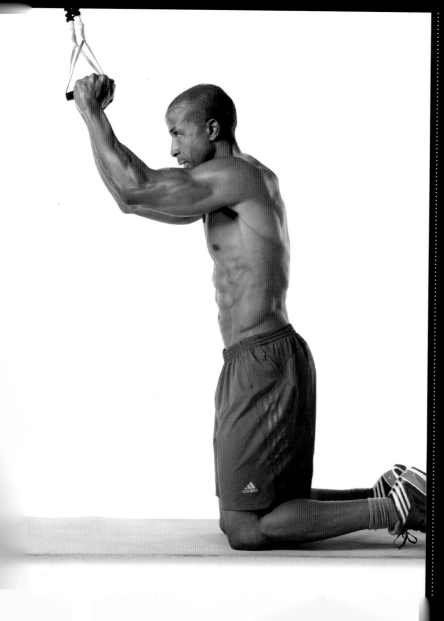

START
Fasten a resistance band above you (for example, at the top of a door or on a door handle) and kneel on the ground, keeping your thighs, torso, and head in a straight line. Hold the ends of the resistance bands in front of your head with your hands wide enough to cradle your face.

BEGINNER

Use a resistance band with less tension or simply do the movement without any resistance, focusing on the contraction in your upper abs.

ADVANCED

Add more tension by using a tighter resistance band and bring the contraction further down so your elbows almost touch the ground (see bottom photo below).

ACTION

Crunch your upper body downward toward the floor, but don't use your arms to extend the resistance band.

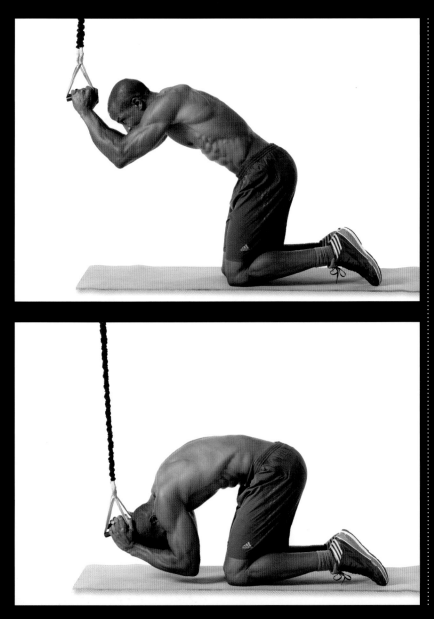

9. CABLE CRUNCH

The cable station in your gym is the busiest for a reason: It works for just about any body part—especially your core.

BEGINNER

To make this move a little easier, lessen the weight on the cable station. If you can't curl the weight with one hand, it's too much. Select a weight that is light for a single arm movement. You'll think it's too light for the contraction, but because you'll be doing this to failure, you'll be building muscle with each rep.

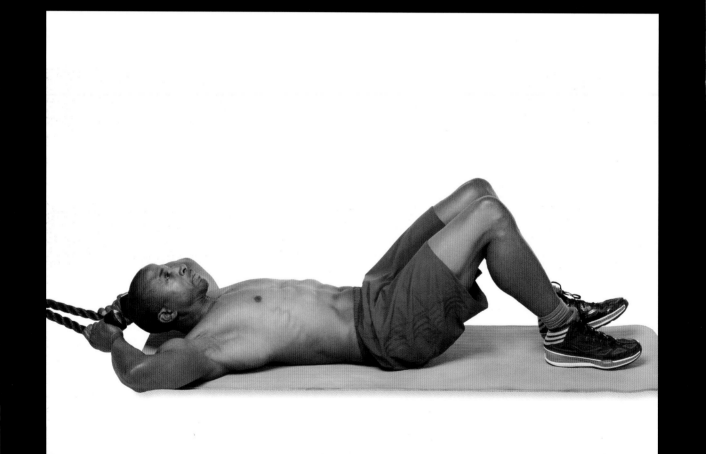

START Lie flat in the typical crunch position with your head 2 feet (61cm) away from the base of a vertical cable station. Hold

ADVANCED

Add intensity to this movement by performing your reps on a Bosu ball and also adding weight.

NOTE
Selecting a weight for any variation of this movement can be difficult. While each step has a benchmark to help you choose an appropriate weight, only you know which weight is right for you after trying the exercise. We advise that you start lighter than you would initially expect. Master the contraction and gradually increase your weight.

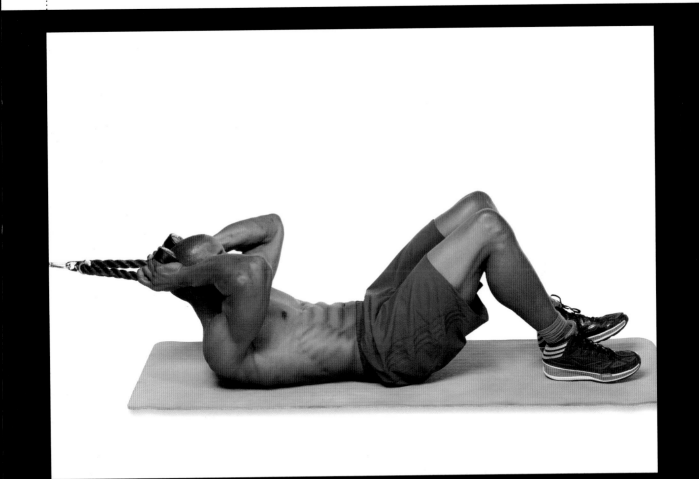

ACTION Crunch your upper torso forward while keeping your arms bent. The movement is only a few inches, but the contraction will be exclusively in the upper abs; do not pull the weight with your arms or use momentum to swing through your reps.

10. DECLINE BENCH CURL UP

A decline bench can be a great tool for building strength in your upper abs because it adds gravity to your contraction. Be sure to select a bench with leg pads so you don't accidentally slide off the bench.

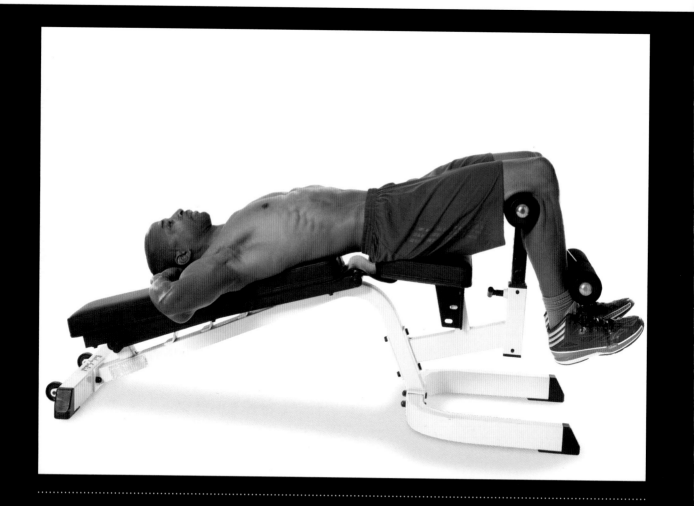

START Lie flat on the decline bench, with your legs tucked around the leg pads so you don't slip off. Put your hands behind your head, cradling your skull. Press your spine flat against the bench.

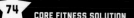

BEGINNER

Because this is an advanced move, there is little that can be done to lessen the intensity. If you attempt this move and it is beyond your fitness level, the most you can expect is to perform partial reps. While this is not recommended, there is still benefit in doing partial reps, but remember not to use momentum or pull with your arms.

ADVANCED

If you've mastered this movement and want to add intensity, we recommend holding a weight plate, dumbbell or kettlebell over your chest at the start of your reps and pressing it up and above your head at the top of each movement.

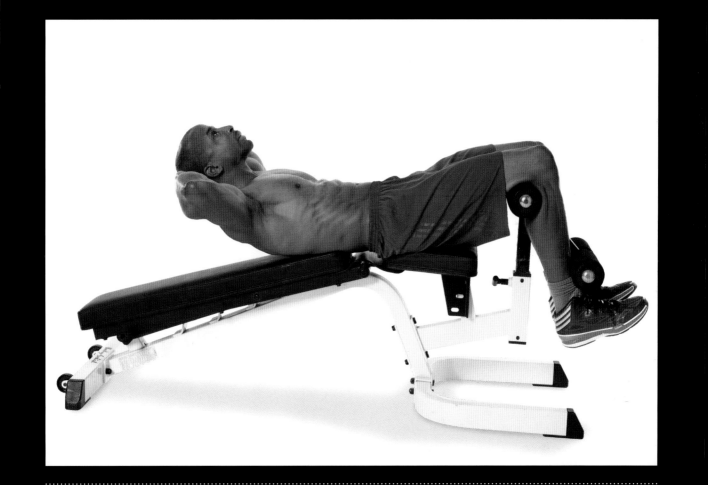

ACTION Curl your upper torso forward, being careful not to pull your head and neck forward for momentum. Your shoulders, middle back,

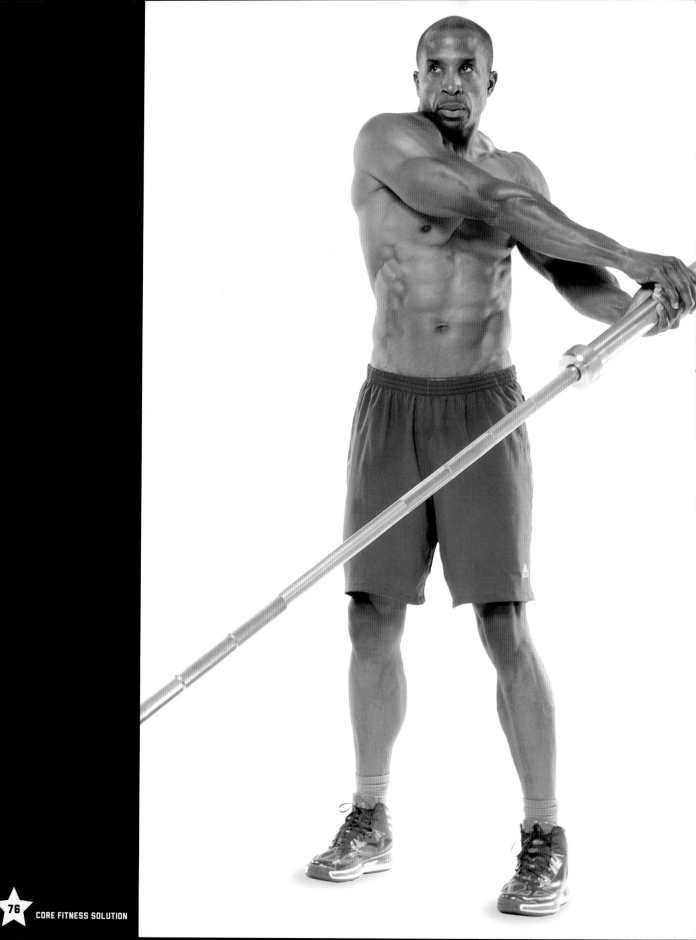

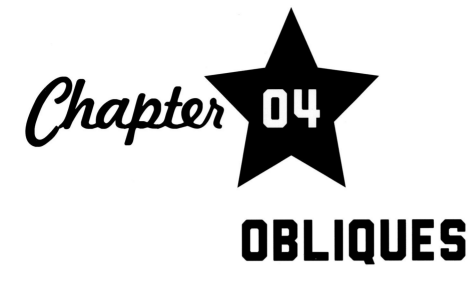

Chapter 04

OBLIQUES

EVER SEE A SERIOUSLY RIPPED FITNESS MODEL'S SIDE TORSO? YOU KNOW, THE AREA ON BOTH SIDES OF THE SIX-PACK? REMEMBER SEEING A COLLECTION OF SLASHED MUSCLES STREAMING FROM THE SIDES OF THAT AREA? THOSE ARE OBLIQUES. BUT IF YOU THINK OBLIQUES ARE JUST A COLLECTION OF LUMPS ON THE SIDES OF SERIOUSLY FIT OR THIN PEOPLE, YOU'D BE WRONG.

Your obliques are integral to any bending or twisting motion you do. Before you pull out an old bodybuilding magazine to count the obliques, you should know that even though they look like a collection of small muscles on both sides of your core, they're really made up of two muscles: the external obliques (that's the rippling section you can see) and the internal obliques (which you can't really see but, trust us, they're just as important). The external obliques are just under your skin and are arguably the strongest of all your core muscles.

The internal obliques lie between your external obliques and the transversus abdominis.

Why are the obliques important? Do you think you could drive a car very far if you couldn't ever make a turn? Could a baseball player hit a home run without twisting his torso? Could you run, walk, or even turn over in bed if your body couldn't bend? Believe it, they're that important to so many basic movements that we take for granted—and for some folks, they're also a great indicator of your fitness level.

1. SIDE PLANK

You're no stranger to this exercise if you've been doing the tests in the first chapter. If you skipped it, prepare for an intense oblique assault from this simple exercise that fatigues your entire core and overall stamina.

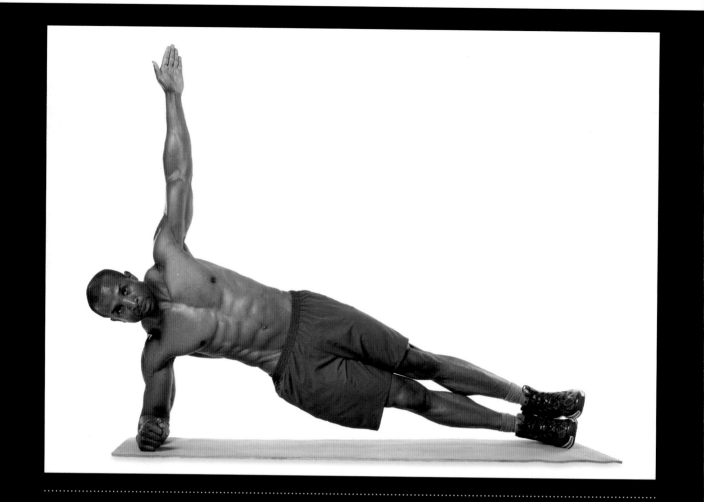

START Balance yourself so only your right foot, right forearm and right fist are holding all your weight. Stretch your left arm above you, pointing to the ceiling.

BEGINNER

If you want to make this move a little easier at the start or even partway through, you can balance yourself on your bottom knee to reduce the intensity.

ADVANCED

Get more out of this plank variation by raising your non-weight-bearing leg in addition to your arm (see photo below).

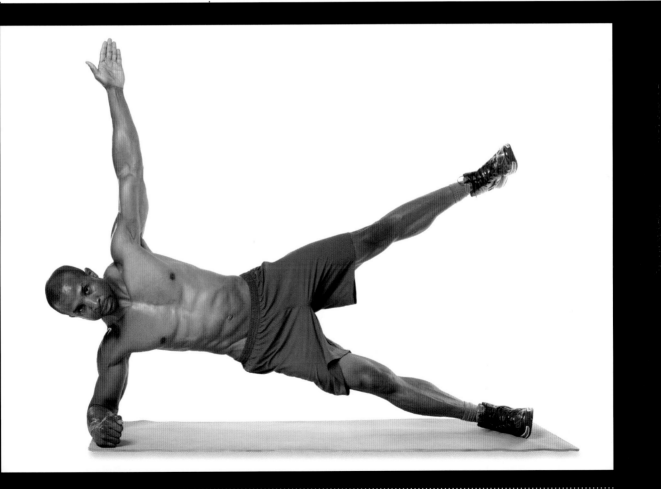

ACTION Hold the pose for as long as you can.

2. SIDE BEND

There's nothing simpler than standing on your two feet and crunching side to side, right? Wrong! In fact, even the most seasoned trainers often do this exercise incorrectly. It's not about how much weight you can carry in your hands, or how much weight you can curl with your biceps. Instead, it's about how much weight your obliques can move from a standing bend position. Sure, you could cheat through this one and swing the weight around and pretend that you hit your obliques. Or you could go light, steady, and meticulous and increase your power exponentially. Your call.

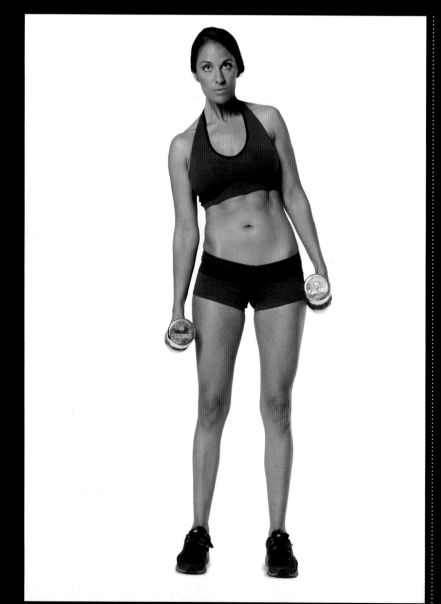

START
Stand with your feet shoulder-width apart, holding a dumbbell in each hand at your sides.

BEGINNER

Try perfecting the movement without weights if you're just getting the hang of this exercise.

ADVANCED

Raise and fully extend your arms so the weights are above your head and parallel to the ceiling. Perform the reps while focusing on your oblique power to create the movement.

ACTION

Bend on one side by lowering your shoulder while contracting your obliques and return to the start. Repeat on both sides.

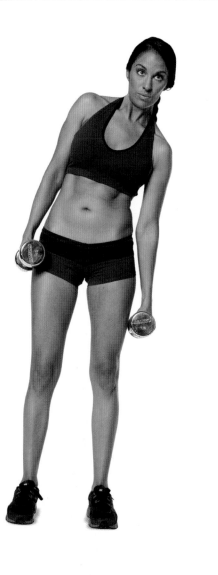

3. STABILITY BALL HIP ROLLS

Quite possibly the safest stability ball exercise you'll find, this move is one that tests your patience and oblique strength with each repetition. Because it's a seemingly easy exercise, it frequently gets rushed through. Our challenge to you is to really focus on your form in this movement and let the power of your core—especially your obliques—take control. When you're done, and inevitably exhausted, you're already on the floor, so you can relax. Thank us later.

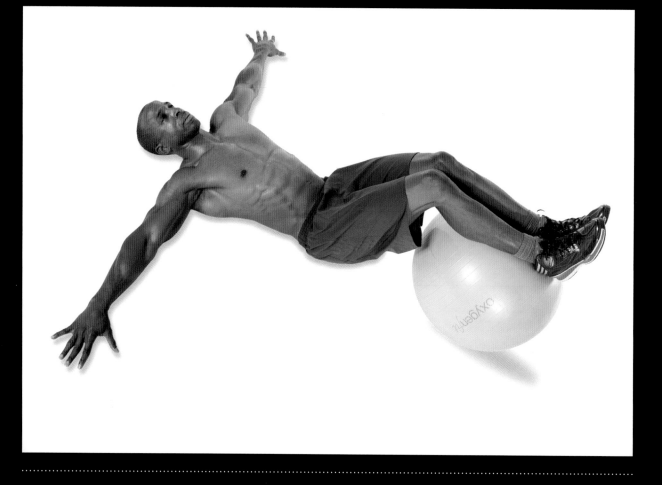

START Lie flat on your back, resting your calf muscles on a stability ball. Flare your hands out at your sides, palms down.

BEGINNER

If you find the stability ball cumbersome in this movement, try doing it without it so your knees are bent at 90 degrees and you move them side to side as previously described.

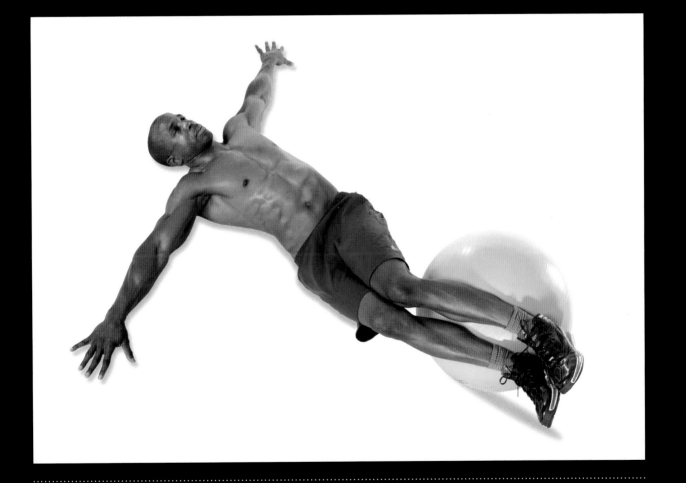

ACTION Slowly move your lower body to the left, allowing your lower torso to twist in the process, but do not raise yourself off the ground. Your left thigh will create a 45-degree angle with the floor at the end of the contraction. Return to the starting position and repeat the motion on the opposite side. Do not swing your legs around on this exercise.

3. STABILITY BALL HIP ROLLS (CONTINUED)

ADVANCED
Increase the depth of your lead leg
from 45 degrees to 90 degrees. You can
also add ankle weights to this move to
increase intensity. Additionally, you can
pulse one side for three reps from the top
to count as one rep.

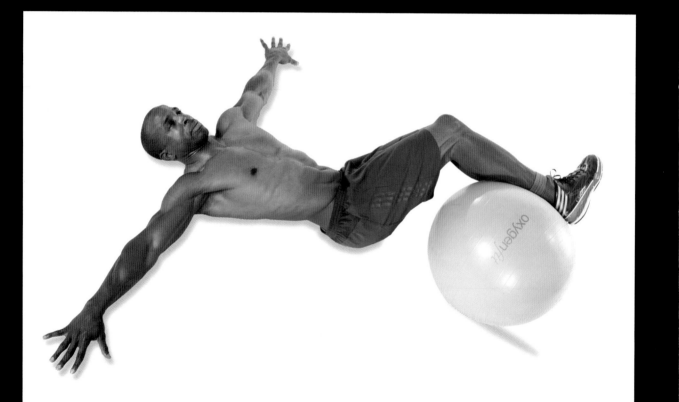

4. BICYCLE CRUNCH

Despite what's implied by the title of this exercise, you won't be using a bicycle. Instead, you'll be on the floor, crunching in two different directions to really harness the power of your obliques. If you're actually a cyclist or just a casual rider, you'll find that this move improves your ability on just about any bike at any speed.

BEGINNER
If you find this move too difficult, you can start with your heels on a bench so you don't have to perform the full range of motion with your legs.

ADVANCED
Add ankle weights to this move to make it harder.

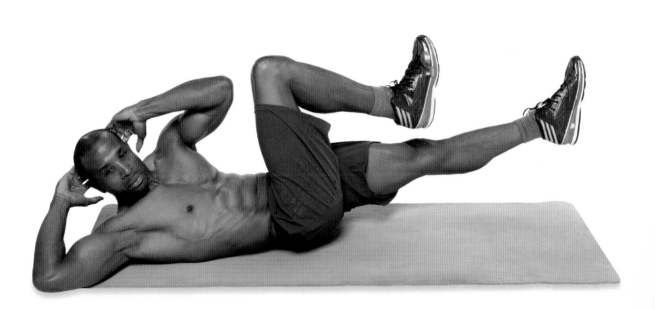

START Lie flat in a crunch position with

ACTION Crunch your upper body forward and to the side

5. CROSS BODY CRUNCH

This move is a variation on the basic crunch you fell in love (or hate) with in the previous chapters and focuses on your sides.

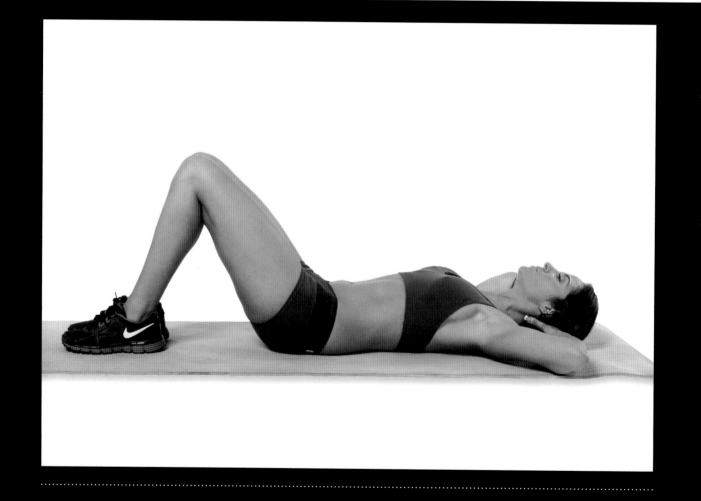

START Lie on the floor in a standard crunch position, with your feet flat on the floor and your hands behind your head.

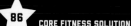

BEGINNER

If you're finding this exercise too difficult, try performing partial reps until you can master the full movement.

ADVANCED

Kick up the intensity by lifting your legs off the ground so your calf muscles are parallel to the ground and your toes are pointing straight up to the ceiling.

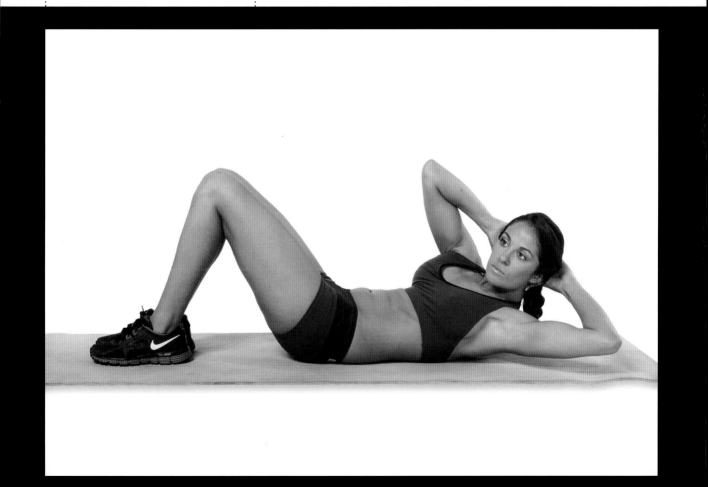

ACTION Crunch forward and across so your right elbow comes up over your torso. Keep your

6. SEATED BROOM TWIST

You really don't need much to do this exercise. If you think it'll be easy, though, you're obliques will tell you otherwise. Get comfortable on a less than plush seat with a broomstick over your shoulders and results will follow.

BEGINNER

Because this is one of the easier movements in this chapter, there is little more you can do to make it less challenging other than to perform partial reps and gradually get better over time. If that's still too much, try doing the movement without the broomstick.

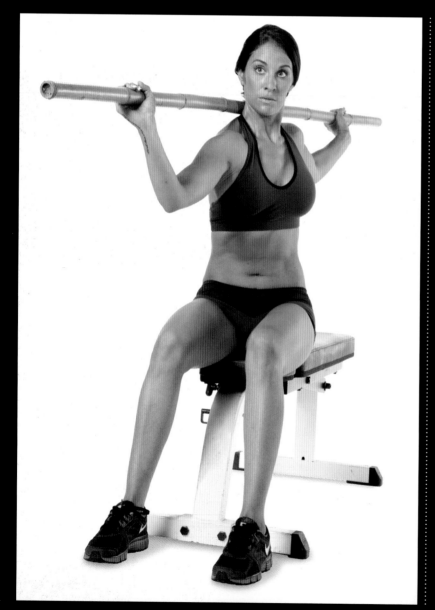

START

Sit on the edge of a bench or similarly padded surface with your feet flat on the floor. Rest a broomstick across your neck, above your shoulders, with your hands holding either side and your elbows bent at 45 degrees.

ADVANCED

If you still want to tackle this move and are itching to increase the intensity, hold the contraction for three counts at the end of the movement and then crunch your torso forward on that side, bringing that end of the broomstick just above your knees. Still want more? Stand in an isometric lunge and twist. Switch feet after one side is tired, but count reps or track time to produce even work on both sides.

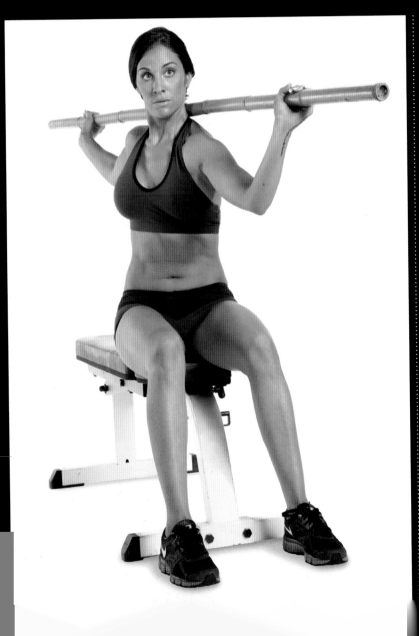

ACTION

Twist your torso to each side, making sure not to pull with your arms. Squeeze your abdominals with control at the end of each twist. Use the stick as a barometer for your balance and to ensure that you do not hunch or bend forward.

7. STABILITY BALL OBLIQUE CRUNCH

Almost every oblique crunch requires a twisting motion of your torso. The stability ball oblique crunch, however, is one of very few crunches that actually forces you to crunch with your obliques in a linear movement instead of across your body.

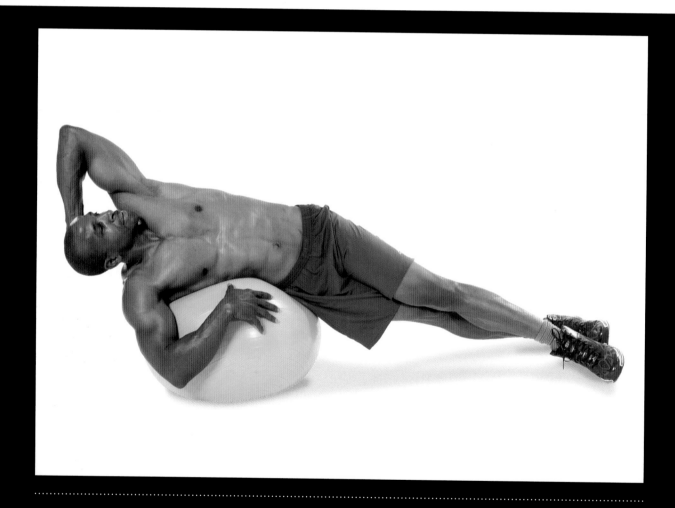

START Steady yourself on a stability ball so your side (armpit to hip) is the only part of your body touching the ball. Stretch out your legs and place your feet on their sides or against a wall for better balance. If your right side is on the ball, your left arm will be up by your head, bent at the elbow so your hand can cradle your skull.

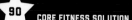

BEGINNER

If you're finding that you can't balance yourself on the stability ball and perform your reps, use a Bosu ball.

ADVANCED

If you want to add intensity to this movement, point the arm that is bent by your head straight up throughout the movement.

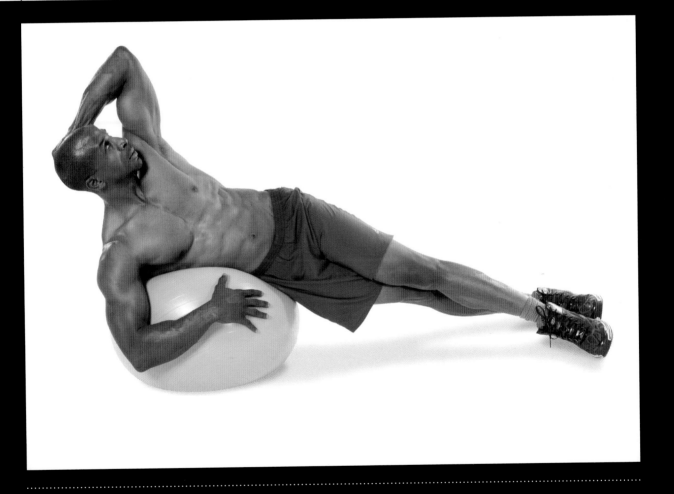

ACTION Crunch your upper body off the ball toward your legs using your obliques to perform the movement. Repeat on both sides.

8. HANGING LEG RAISES WITH TWISTS

Much like the hanging leg raise in chapter 2, this variation is great for overall core strength but places more emphasis on your obliques.

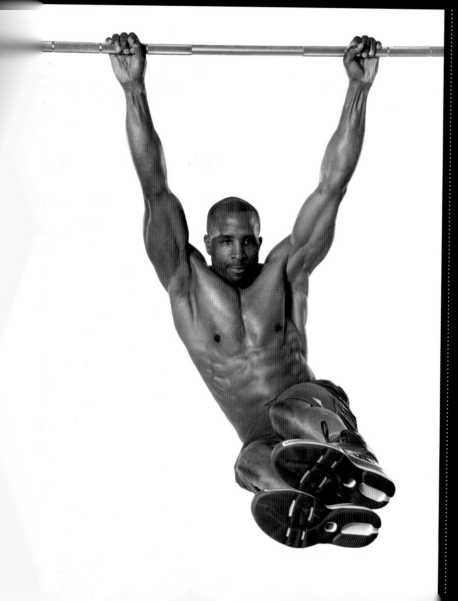

BEGINNER

Make this move easier by performing partial reps. Remember not to jerk your weight to perform your reps.

ADVANCED

Add ankle weights or resistance bands to up the intensity of this move.

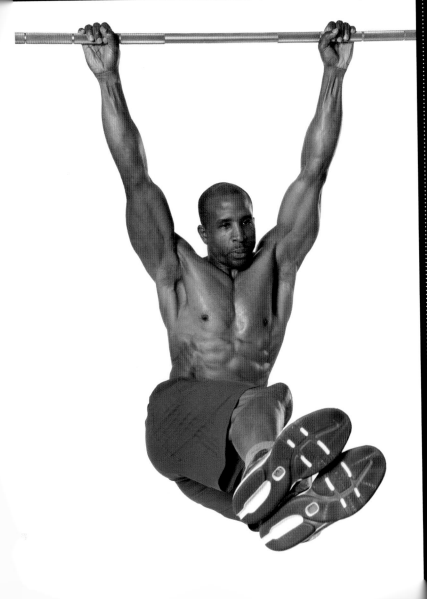

ACTION

Crunch your legs up toward your torso and twist your legs to the side, creating a crunching motion on your obliques. Do not bring your knees past your hips and continue looking straight ahead throughout the movement. Slowly return your legs to the starting position without using momentum. Repeat on both sides.

9. LANDMINES

As a general rule, it's probably best not to announce that you're working on some landmines. Language notwithstanding, adding landmines to your core workout is a great way to target your obliques. Some gyms have a landmine apparatus that allows you to attach an Olympic bar so there can be no shifting, but we prefer just using the corner in any room of your house. For those who don't have a bar at home, or simply don't want to start with that weight, you can still perform the movement with any broom or even a hockey stick. As a bonus, if you're a hockey player, you'll be glad to know that this exercise will do more to improve your performance than your last game of pick-up with your pals. How? The twisting motion will help with your strides and shot follow-through.

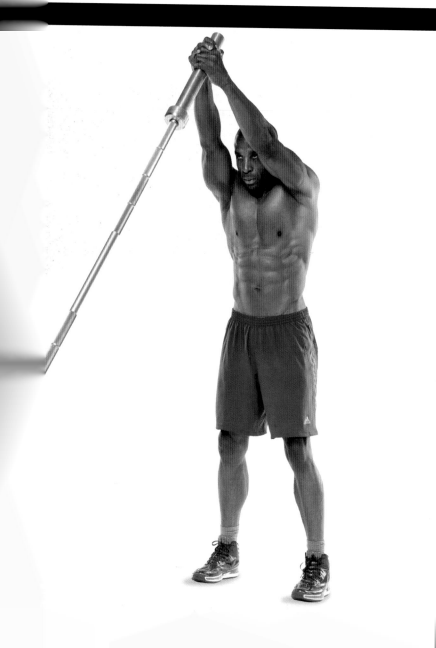

START

Rest a weight bar in a corner, angled up. Stand with your feet shoulder-width apart about 5 feet (1.5m) from the corner and grip the bar near the top with your hands. You can interlace your fingers if it allows for a more secure grip.

BEGINNER

If an Olympic bar is too heavy, try using a broom or a hockey stick.

ADVANCED

If you're using a weighted bar, you can add a weight plate to the top of the bar to provide more intensity to each rep.

ACTION

Slowly lower the bar from directly over your head to the left, letting your left arm come down to your side and your right arm cross your body. Repeat on your right side. Do not simply move the weight with your arm strength. Instead, lock your arms straight and engage your core. Focus on the very minor motion within your core to allow the movement to happen.

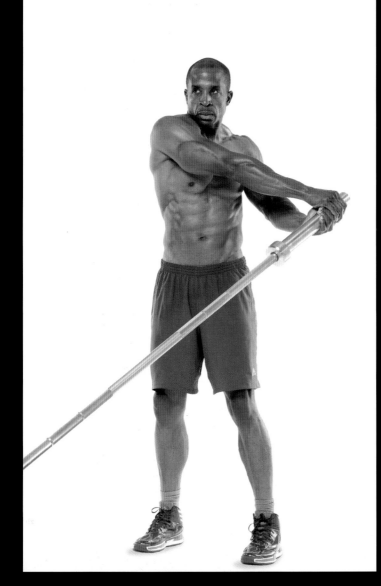

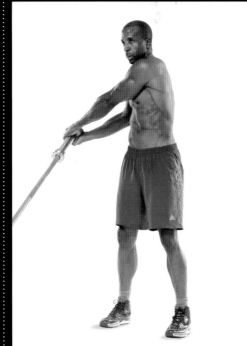

10. KNEELING CABLE OBLIQUE CRUNCH

Most pulling motions from this position will focus on your upper abs and the initial crunching motion of this move will affect on that part of your midsection. The key for your obliques is the twisting motion that follows as you lower the weight even further across your body. If you want to skip the gym, you can do this move with an exercise band affixed to the top of a door.

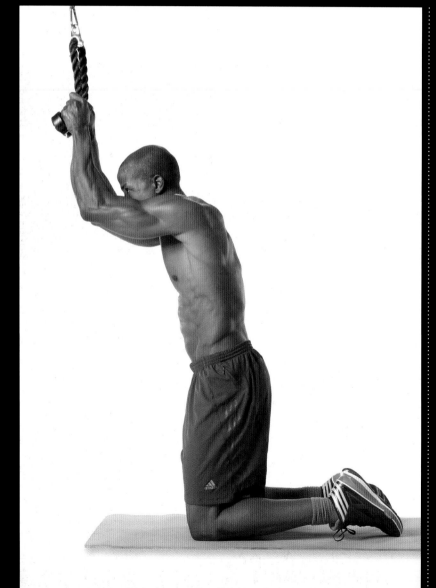

START
Kneel at a cable station with the cable set at the top. Set up the rope attachment and lower it down to you with both hands. Maintain a 90-degree bend in your arms and place your knees shoulder-width apart.

BEGINNER

If this move is too difficult for you, lower the weight you've selected or simply perform each rep with no weight at all to master the motion of each rep.

ADVANCED

Add more weight to this move to make it more difficult. You can also raise the knee that your elbow is twisting toward to create a double crunch motion. Do not lift your knee more than a couple of inches off the ground.

ACTION

Crunch your torso down toward the floor while twisting, so your right elbow goes just in front of your left knee, making sure not to touch the floor. Alternate on both sides.

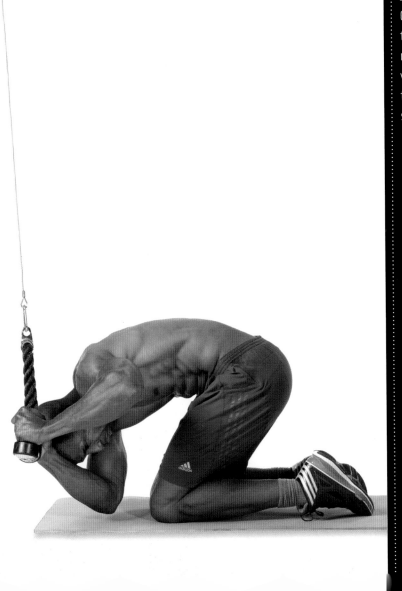

11. CAPTAIN'S CHAIR SIDE LEG LIFT

The captain's chair might just be one of the few apparatuses that make going to a physical gym to train your abs worth it. However, most people use this apparatus incorrectly when attempting to work their abdominal muscles. You really can't mimic the movements you can do in this chair unless you have a parallel bar setup. Our advice: Hit the chair when you go to the gym and choose a core workout that's packed with gym-friendly moves.

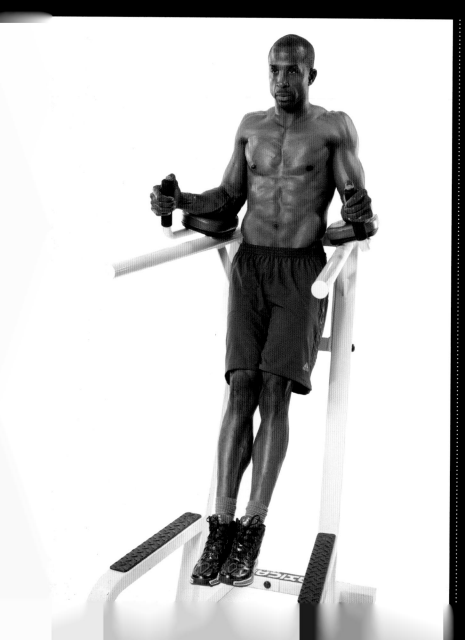

START
Stand in the captain's chair with your back firmly against the back pad and your forearms on the hand pads. Hold the front handles to ensure you don't slip. Your feet should be dangling freely above the floor without any obstruction. Most importantly, do not let your feet go under your hips. Keep them positioned slightly in front of you during the downward motions of the exercise while keeping your legs together.

BEGINNER

If you can't manage to perform many reps, performing partial reps is an option to make this move easier. You can also try lifting only one leg at a time.

ADVANCED

To really pick up the intensity of this exercise, instead of simply raising your legs and bending your knees, kick your legs out and do twisting circles as you lower back to the start position.

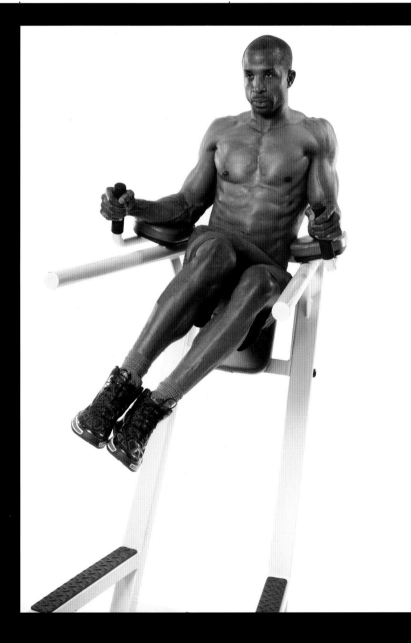

ACTION

Crunch your legs up while bending your knees. Twist your legs to either side using the power of your lower abs and obliques. Repeat on both sides.

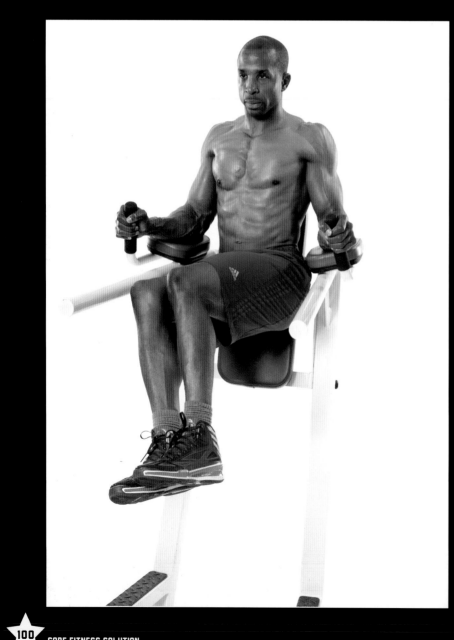

HINT

Are your shoulders feeling a little jammed up after doing this move? You're probably cheating or not aligning properly in the chair. Don't let your traps sink or your shoulders come together. No slouching either! Also, if you're whipping your legs up and down to do a rep, those don't count. Sorry!

12. OBLIQUE CRUNCH WITH LEGS UP

Who says you can't get a workout when you're lying down? All you need to make this exercise target your sides and build core strength is a flat surface and the time to go to failure on each set. Enjoy.

BEGINNER
Make this move easier by performing partial reps or by leaving your legs flat on the floor.

ADVANCED
Add ankle weights to kick up the intensity of this move.

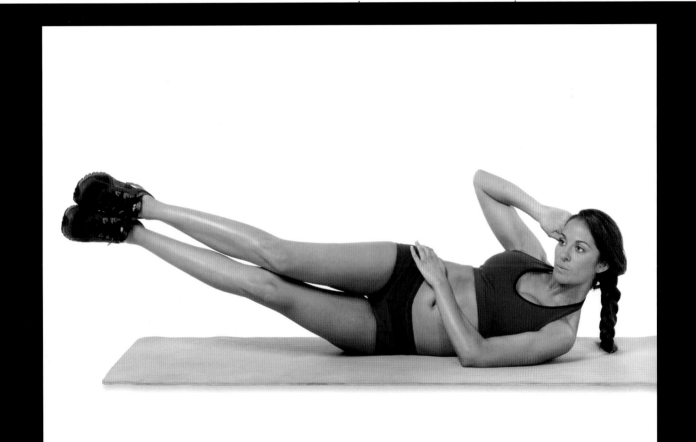

START Lie on your side with your feet together and the arm closer to the ceiling bent and cradling your head. Place your other arm at your side, bent upward so your hand is resting on your hip.

ACTION Crunch your legs up toward your torso while crunching your upper body down toward your legs. This double crunching motion will work your obliques with minimal movement so you don't have to raise your hip or ribs off the floor to complete a rep. Repeat on both sides.

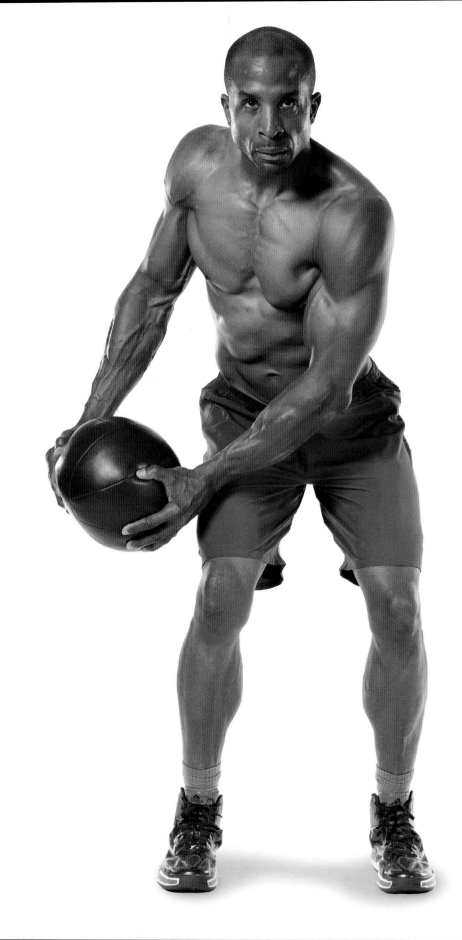

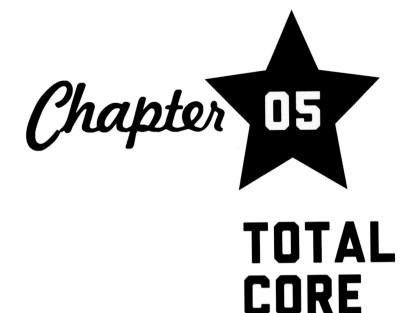

Chapter 05

TOTAL CORE

WE PROMISED YOU A TOTAL CORE SOLUTION, AND WHILE ALL THE PREVIOUS CHAPTERS ARE INTEGRAL TO FULFILLING THAT PROMISE, YOU REALLY CAN'T GET TO YOUR FULL CORE POTENTIAL WITHOUT APPROACHING IT FROM A 360-DEGREE, ALL-INCLUSIVE LINE OF ATTACK. WHAT WILL THAT TRANSLATE TO YOU AS THE TRAINER IN THIS CHAPTER?

Fewer crunches and less of what's more commonly out there for six-pack development but with more core stability and overall core strength moves. You may have never seen many of these exercises, and if you have, you may have thought they were, well, bunk. But the truth of total core development is in this chapter. And it comes in the form of more complex contractions, greater burst speed movements, far more challenging balancing actions and, ultimately, some of the most advanced exercises that you've likely ever tried.

At this point in your exercise selections, you've already targeted all the muscles that show and some of the ones that don't. Now it's time to take the great-looking sports car you've designed that can turn on a dime, as well as push, pull and brace like an industrial truck, and give it the engine that will have you performing better at every single movement you make from now on.

1. PLANK

You should be a master at this move already if you've been following the testing outlined in chapter 1. If not, we suggest you go back and test your core now before trying to jump into these workouts. The plank is arguably the best barometer for your core strength and should be a staple of almost any core workout.

BEGINNER

If you're just starting out, try making this move with your knees down.

ADVANCED

Try kicking this up a notch with any of the variations listed in the test section. Our suggestion is the arm and leg raise combination.

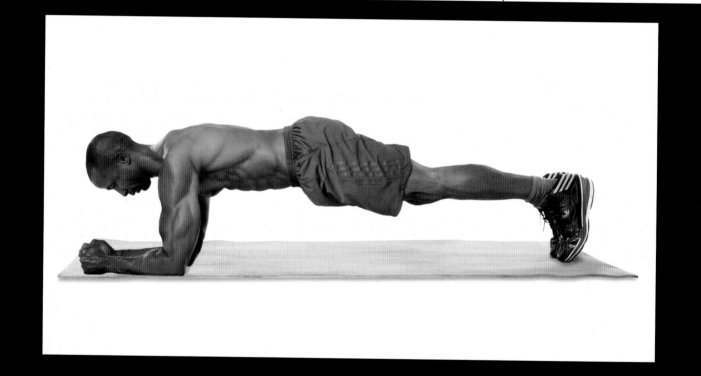

START Lie face down on a mat so your toes, forearms and fists are holding all of your weight off the ground. Your body should create a straight, plank-like figure. Create a neutral (flat) spine by tilting your pelvis forward. Engage your abdominals, glutes and thigh muscles. Your butt and hips should stay in this same line; make sure they don't sag or rise beyond the level. Do not round your shoulders. Maintain this position throughout while looking straight down at your hands.

ACTION Simply hold this position for as long as you can without breaking form.

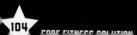

VARIATION: PUSH-UP PLANK

Since the plank is such an important move to your core strength and stability, there are many variations you can try. To target more muscles in your body and further enhance your strength and core stability, we suggest altering the plank starting position into a push-up. Perform one push-up and at the bottom of the repetition, then hold as you would with a plank. This is a way to do the plank as reps instead of continuous hold as described above.

VARIATION: WALKING PLANK

You can also try walking planks. Move from a regular plank into a push-up plank by lifting each arm one at a time and then returning to the regular plank position one arm at a time. Do not let your hips swing side to side and remain in a strong plank throughout the movement.

2. SPIDERMANS

Ever want to be a superhero? Would you settle for superhero abs? This movement mimics the motion that Spiderman makes while crawling walls—except you're on the ground throughout. Don't worry: The Green Goblin will be sitting this one out.

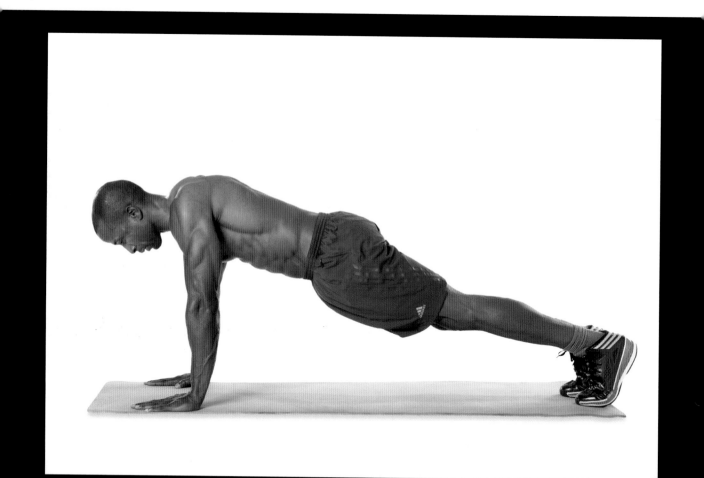

START Start in a standard push-up position with your hands flat on the floor and your feet hip-width apart.

ACTION As you lower your body in the push-up, bring your left knee forward until it reaches your left elbow, then place it back next to the other foot and finish the push-up by returning to the starting position. For the next push-up, switch sides.

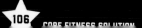

BEGINNER

If you want to make this move easier, do the entire exercise balancing your weight on your knees.

ADVANCED

Kick up the intensity by bringing your left knee to your right elbow in the starting position, alternating on both sides (see bottom photo below).

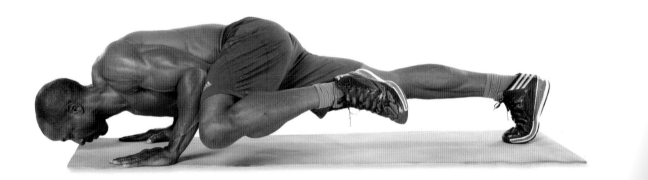

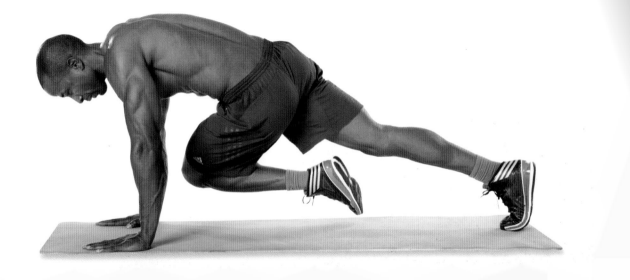

3. MOUNTAIN CLIMBERS

This may look like a standard push-up gone wrong, but the running-like movement of your legs while retaining a stable core will really target your abs. You can do this move from anywhere, but you'll need grip to perform it properly. If you're a sprinter or runner of any kind, doing the mountain climber will ensure you're first out of the gate every time.

BEGINNER

If this move is too difficult for you, start in a plank position. This will conserve some strength for the actual movement.

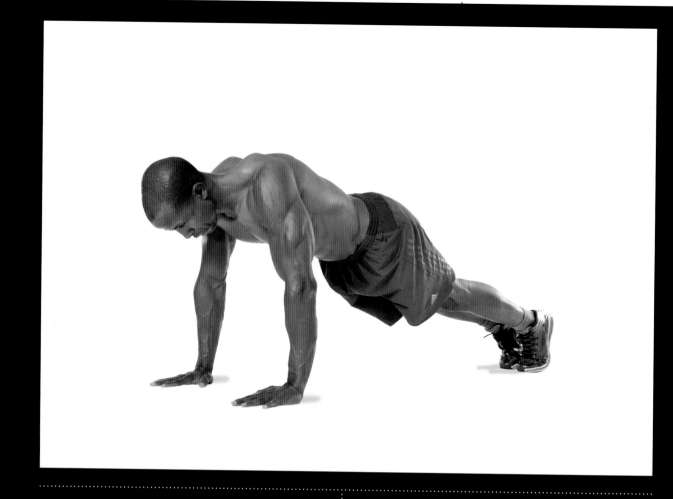

START Get into a standard push-up position with your feet hip-width apart and arms extended.

ACTION Alternate bringing your knees toward your chest as though you were trying to kick up into a sprint. Don't allow your shoulders to round or your upper back to hunch down.

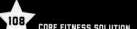

ADVANCED

If you're finding yourself doing a lot of these and want to challenge yourself, try raising your legs diagonally across your chest on each rep for each leg.

MAKE IT A BURPEE

The mountain climber exercise can easily be the precursor to a burpee. Once you've mastered the movement, move both knees toward your chest and then go back to the starting position. From there, gear it up a notch by thrusting up and standing off of the kicking-up motions. From that shoulder-width standing position, jump as high as you can, lifting your arms into the air. This move targets your legs, arms and core, and, when done quickly in succession to failure, it can also be a great cardio workout on its own.

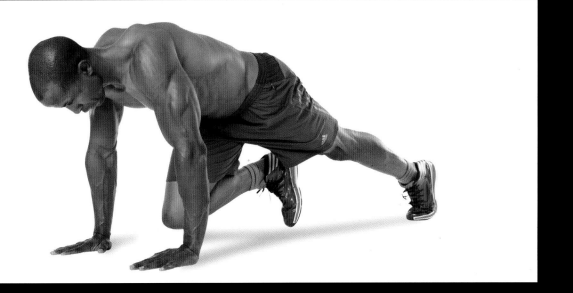

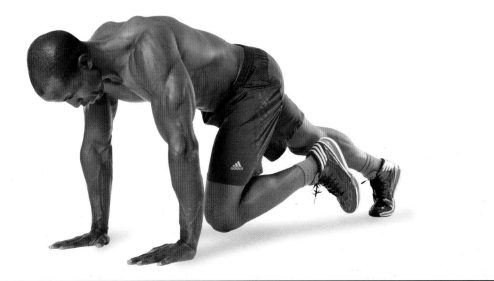

4. DOG POINTERS

Sound silly? Sure. But we're not asking you to simply point out something like your pet might. Instead, this kind of dog pointer will create greater core stability through each precise contraction. You won't need Rover to spot you on this one either.

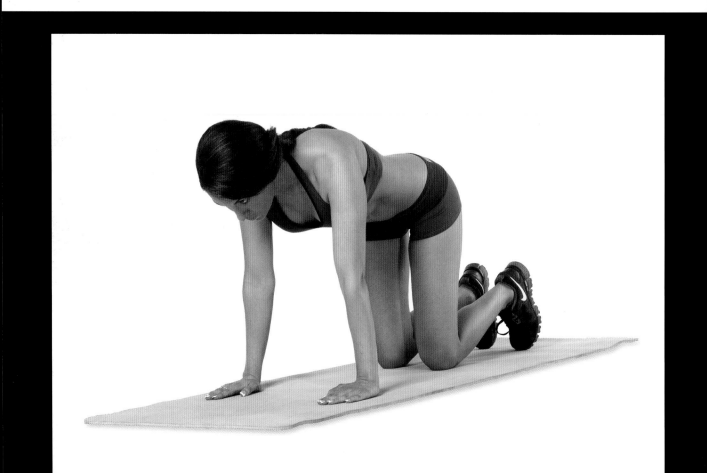

START If you didn't think that the start of this position required you to get on the floor on your hands and knees, you probably didn't read the name of the exercise. Just remember to keep your

BEGINNER

This move is one of the more beginner-friendly choices in the chapter. If you find it too difficult, try raising only an arm or a leg in each rep

ADVANCED

Add ankle weights and light dumbbells (or wrist weights) to make this move a little more challenging.

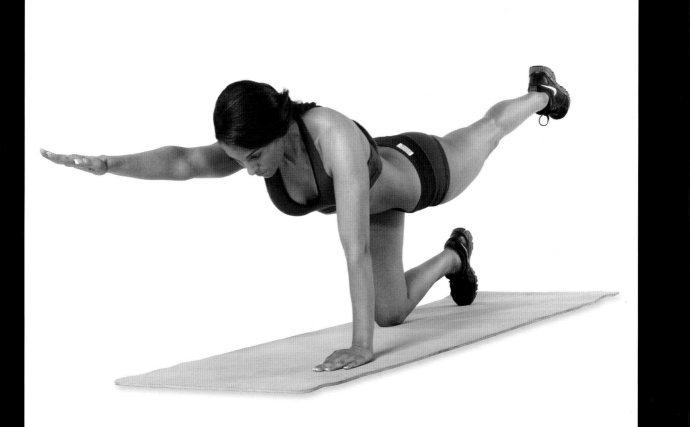

ACTION Extend your right arm forward and your left leg backward to create a straight line with your spine. Focus on making the tips of the fingers on your outstretched arm and the toes in your raised leg extend as far apart as possible. Hold the

5. ROLL-UPS

Looks like a standard crunch? At a glance, it's easy to make that mistake. Perform this move properly and you'll find that the range of motion is coupled with holding back the temptation to help with your hips and legs, forcing you to brace your entire core.

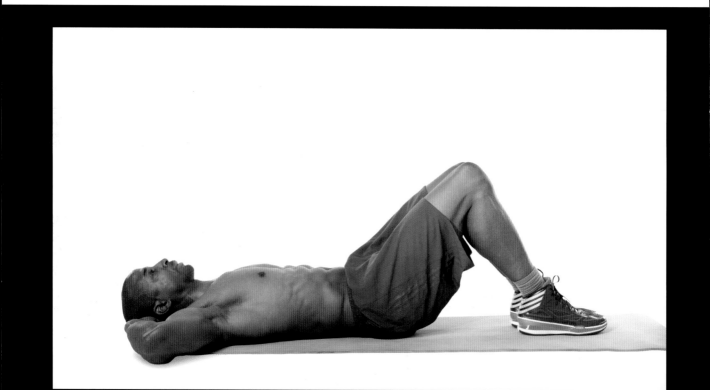

START Lie on a mat in a standard crunch position with your feet flat on the floor, knees bent, and hands behind

ACTION Roll up your upper body so your shoulder blades come off the

BEGINNER

If you find this move too difficult, perform partial reps.

ADVANCED

Make this move harder by rolling straight up, but remember to keep your feet flat on the floor (see bottom photo below).

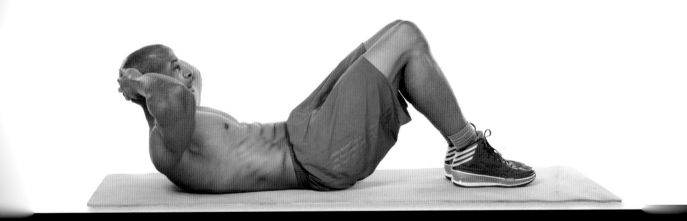

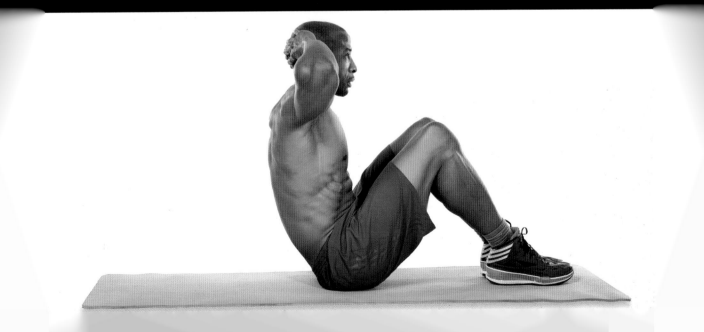

6. STABILITY BALL KNEE TUCK

Targeting your lower abs and your overall core stability, the stability ball knee tuck has a full range of motion, but the final few inches of the movement are the most difficult. When all you want to do is get through your reps without falling off the ball, it's easy to sacrifice your form, but doing fewer reps with proper form is better for your overall core strength and stability.

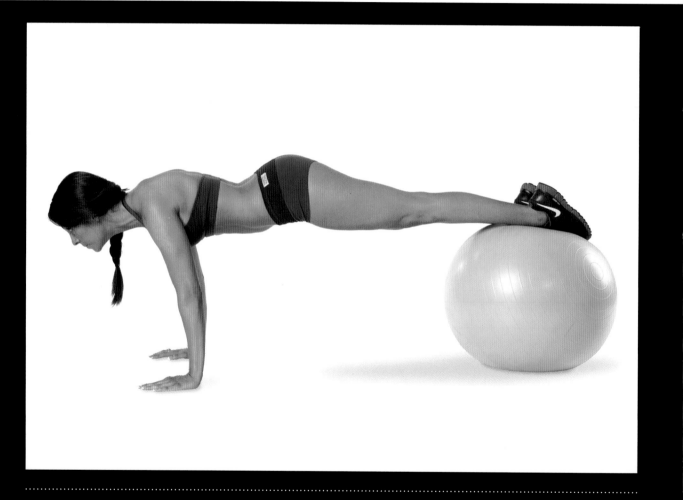

START Get into a push-up position with your feet balanced on a stability ball.

BEGINNER

The stability ball knee tuck is an advanced move and, as such, partial reps may be the only way to perform it with any decreased difficulty. Our advice, if you're going to do partials, is to make sure that you do not allow your butt to rise throughout the movement.

ADVANCED

Get more intense with this move by doing it with alternating legs on the ball.

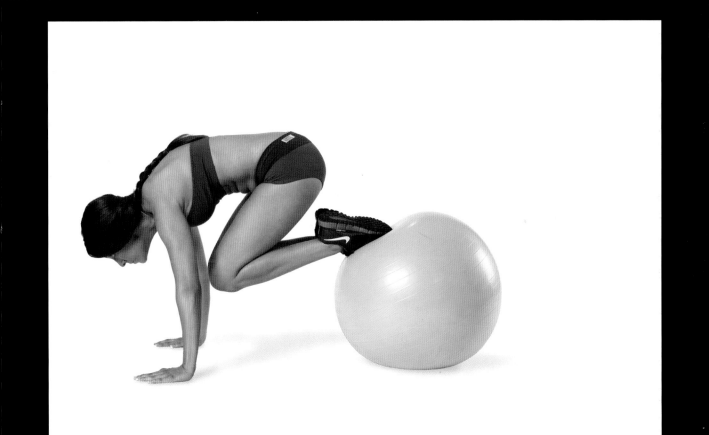

ACTION Crunch your legs in toward your chest, but do not allow your butt to rise up to perform

7. PIKE

Every time you use a stability ball, you have to remember that your core strength is being tested almost as much as any individual muscle. The pike is a great move to enhance your stability and strengthen your core, but adding this move to your repertoire too early could result in injury. We recommend you work on easier moves such as those earlier in this chapter before making this a staple of your workout.

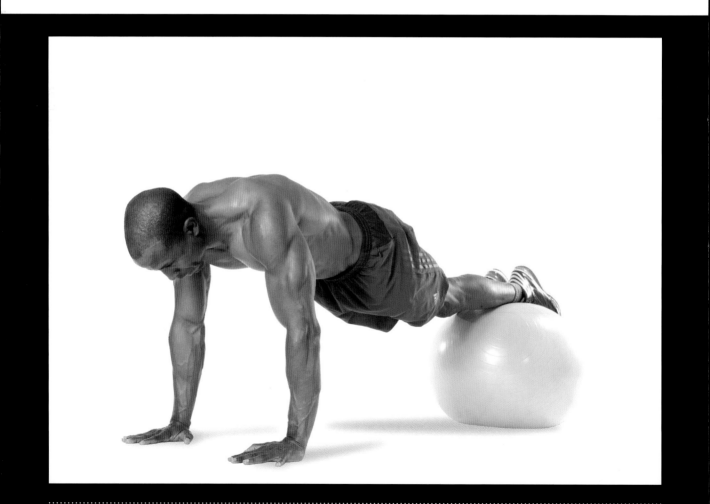

START Get into a push-up position with your feet flat and

BEGINNER

Because this is an advanced move, there's little you can do to make it easier other than to work on your fundamental stability in simpler moves. However, if you want to try the pike but find yourself unable to get it exactly right, focus on doing partial reps.

ADVANCED

Making this move harder isn't wise. The stability it takes to perform each rep should be challenging enough. Focus on the result instead of bragging rights.

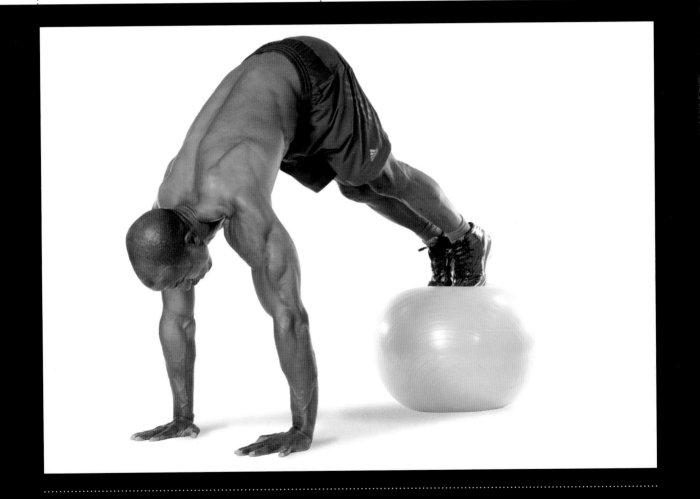

ACTION Raise your pelvis while using your core to bring your legs forward, letting your feet roll in so you end up balancing on your toes. Don't move your arms throughout this exercise and do not let your legs be the driver for the reps. Focus on your core strength to move your body.

8. CABLE PUSH-PULL

It would be easy to think that the twisting motion of this move is where all the core benefits come from, but the truth is that every element of the cable push-pull enhances your overall core strength. This move is great for athletes who have to pivot while running, especially football, hockey, and basketball players.

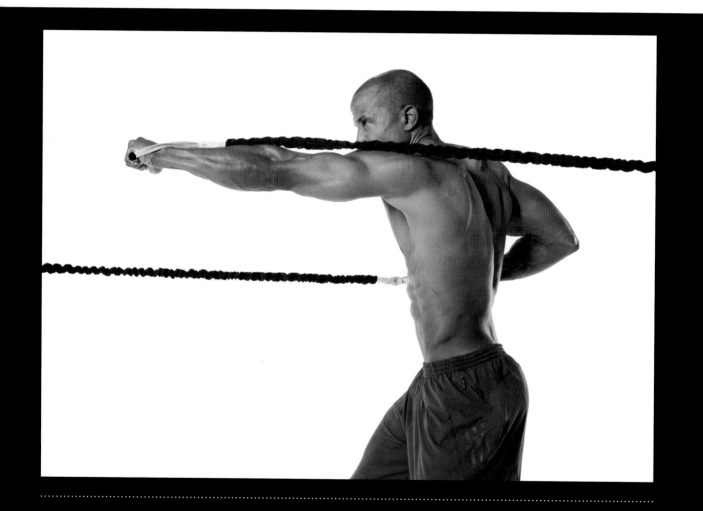

START Attach two D-ring handles to the middle clips of a two-sided cable station. Grab the handles, making sure that the arm extended in front of you (the pull) is straight and the arm behind you (the push) is bent at 90 degrees. Place your right leg a step ahead of your left. Arch your left foot and keep your right foot flat.

BEGINNER

If this move is too difficult for you, try doing the movement with two very light dumbbells in each hand or simply lower the weight at the cable stations.

ADVANCED

Add more weight at the cable stations and focus on not letting your arms do the movement for you to make this move more difficult.

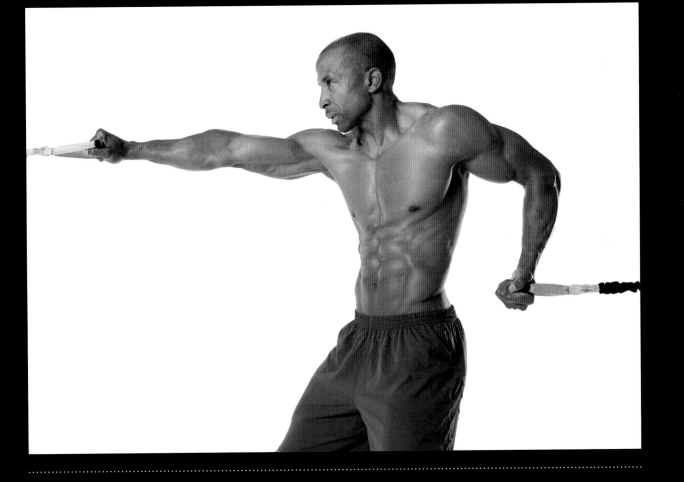

ACTION Pull the cable with your right arm while pushing the cable with your left, keeping your arms at the same level and twisting your torso to complete the movement. Repeat on both sides.

9. CABLE LAWNMOWER

The cable lawnmower is possibly the most functional of all core movements. Aptly titled, it mimics the movement you make when manually starting a lawnmower. Although it is best to do this movement on a cable machine at a gym, you can recreate it with resistance bands or simply with a weight of your choice in your hands.

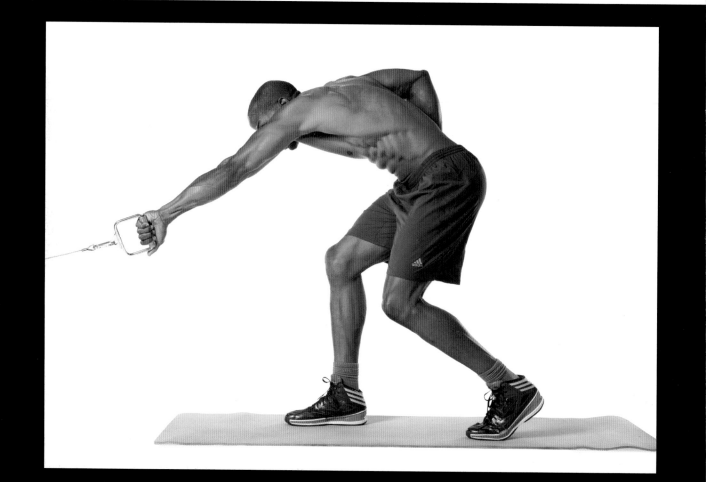

START Attach a D-ring handle to the bottom clip of a cable station. Grab the handle with your left hand, keeping your arm extended and straight. Place your right leg a step ahead of your left in an isometric lunge. Arch your left foot and keep your right foot flat. Remember not to round your shoulders or hunch your back throughout the movement.

BEGINNER

If this move is too difficult for you, lower the weight on the cable station or just perform the movement without any apparatus at all, mastering the motion and contraction through each rep.

ADVANCED

Adding weight to this move will make it more difficult.

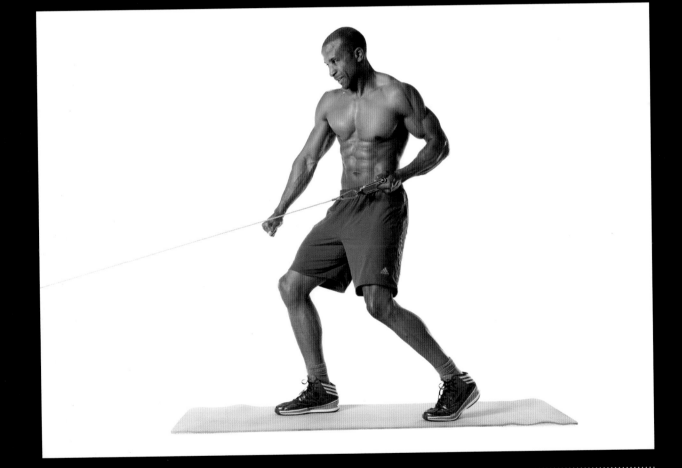

ACTION Pull the handle back while straightening out your stance but maintaining the arch in your left foot. Repeat on both sides.

10. WEIGHTED HIP RAISE ON A BENCH

Quite possibly one of the most versatile movements that targets your core, the weighted hip raise should be a staple of your repertoire. You'll need a bench, couch, chair, or even a staircase to do this move correctly. Although there are variations, we suggest using a bit of padding for your back and shoulders during this movement. Instead of a medicine ball, you can also use a dumbbell or weight plate for extra intensity.

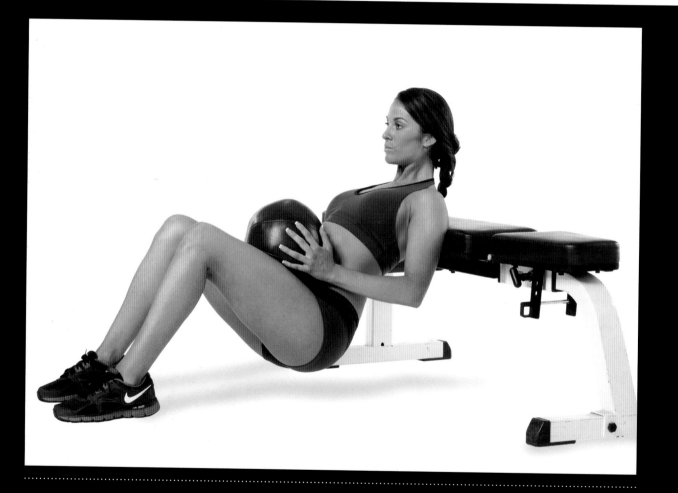

START Balance your shoulders against a bench and place your feet flat on the floor while maintaining a 90-degree angle in your knees. Hold a medicine ball between your thighs.

BEGINNER

If this too difficult for you, try it from a lying down position on the floor.

ADVANCED

Kick it up a notch by doing this move on a stability ball. You may want to start without any weight or medicine ball throughout your first set to make sure you have the stability and core strength to do it without falling off the ball.

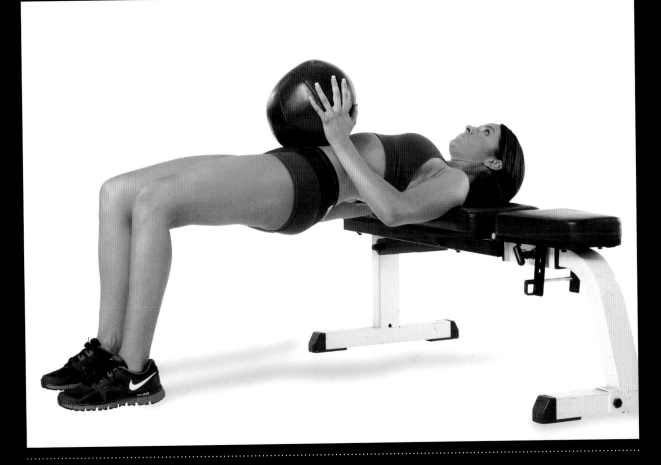

ACTION Thrust your lower body upward by tilting your pelvis (making sure not to use your legs to push the weight). Hold for one count, but remember to keep your body straight and ensure that your hips and butt do not sag.

11. WINDSHIELD WIPERS

This exercise has a simple name for a simple movement that can challenge the strongest cores. The windshield wiper is a precise and meticulous exercise. Remember, you're not in a hurricane—do this move slowly for best results.

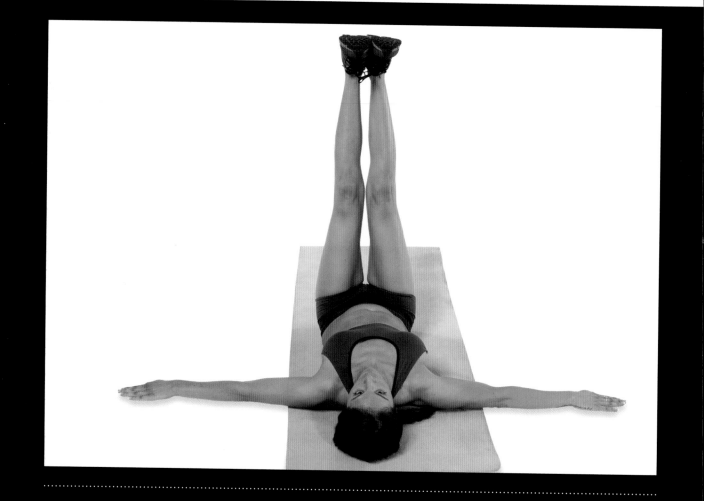

START Lie flat on the floor with your legs together and pointed up so the heels of your feet are parallel to the ceiling. Keep your arms out at your sides.

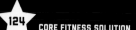

BEGINNER

If you lie on the floor with your legs against the wall so your glutes, hamstrings and heels are touching, you can perform this movement with greater ease.

ADVANCED

If you train with a partner, ask him or her to push your legs down as you're lowering for each rep to make this move more difficult. With each rep, you'll be forced to fight gravity and the extra push from your training partner. You can also increase your speed, but you may have to brace yourself on a fixed area so you don't swing your shoulders and so you maintain good form.

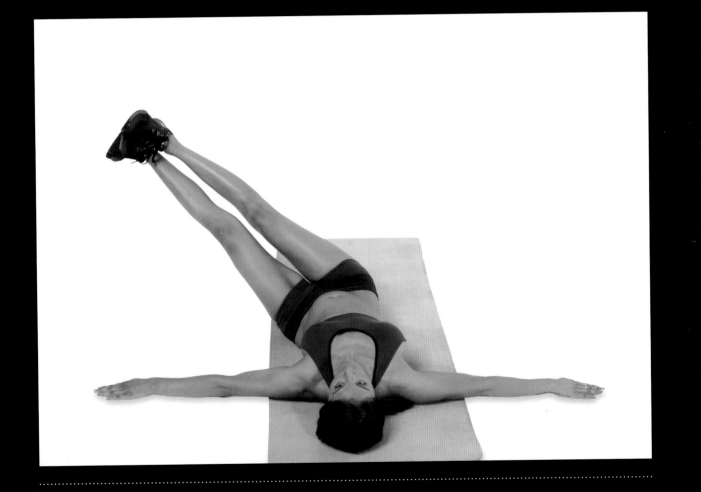

ACTION Bracing your abs throughout the movement, bring your legs down to one side, but keep them together and straight throughout the movement. To finish the rep, return to the starting position and then lower to the other side. Do not swing your legs.

11. WINDSHIELD WIPERS (CONTINUED)

HINT

If you're having difficulty with this move, even with the tip for beginners, try bending your knees, but be sure to keep your knees and feet together throughout the movement.

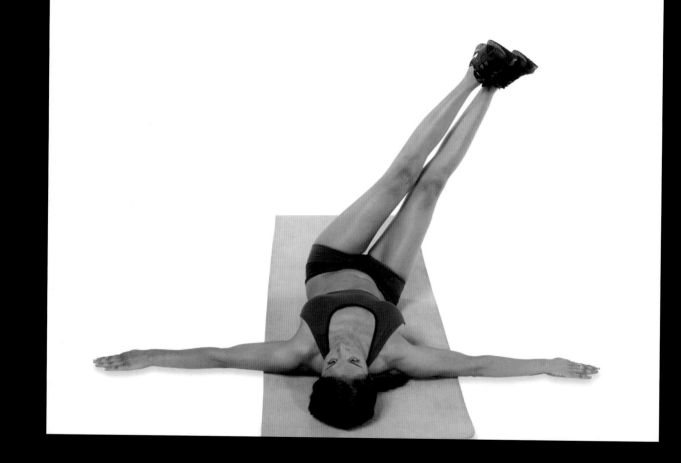

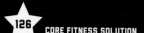

FOCUS

You may not realize it, but keeping your feet together and flat throughout this movement is quite possibly the most important tip for achieving the best results. Why? Because it guides your body and ensures you're not using your feet in any way to help the move. All the power for the movement goes straight to your core.

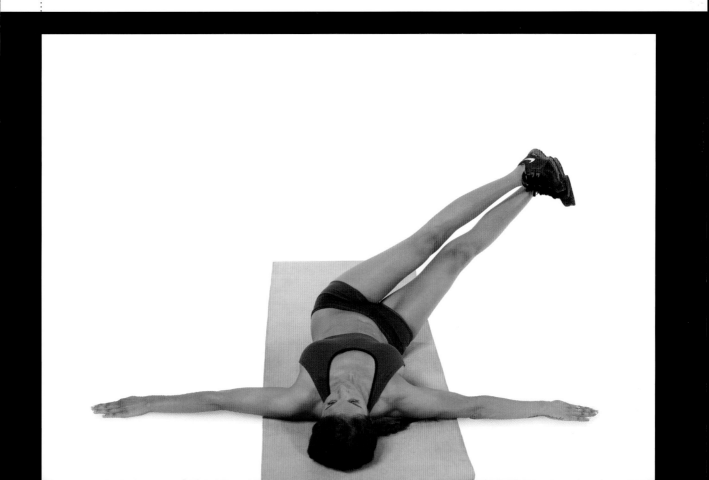

12. MEDICINE BALL FIGURE EIGHT

If you thought medicine balls were solely used as props to make fun of old gyms, you're in for a rude awakening. While the motion of this exercise may not look intense, if you use the power of your core throughout, you'll feel every single nuance through each rep—emphasizing your core strength.

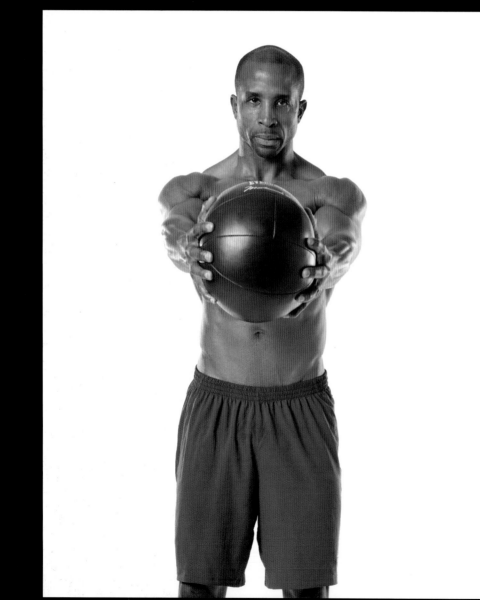

START

Stand with your feet shoulder-width apart holding a medicine ball in your hands directly in front of your chest. Stretch out your arms with a very slight bend in your elbows.

BEGINNER

Doing circles instead of figure eights with the medicine ball will make this move a little easier.

ADVANCED

Make this move a bit more difficult by exaggerating the movement with an even wider motion while making the figure eight.

ACTION

With the power of your core, move the ball in a figure eight in front of you. Perform this movement very meticulously at first. Once you've mastered the motion and feel your core bracing throughout, do it quicker without swinging the ball.

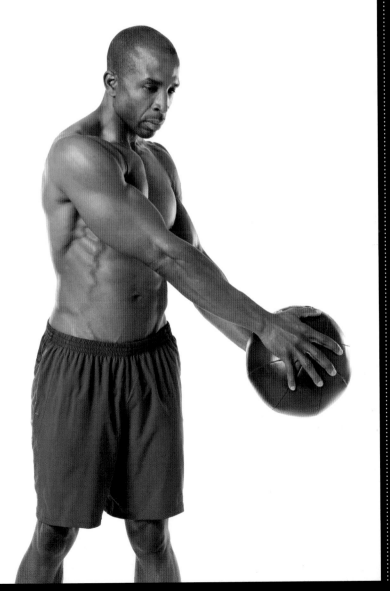

HINT

If you're doing way more reps of this exercise than you are any other in your custom workout, you're probably doing it without harnessing the power of your core. This is one move that is easy to miss the focus on your abs and simply swing through with just your arms doing the work. Think of your arms as dead weight here. All they do is move when your torso moves (through the power of your abs).

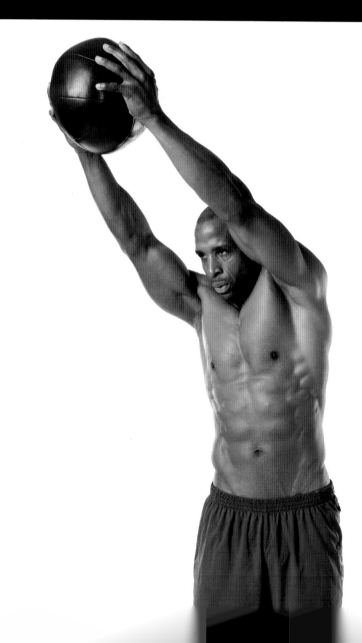

FOCUS
Slow and steady usually is the best course
of action for any exercise. With this one,
however, we suggest speed if you've
mastered the advanced tip. Try doing each rep
as quickly as you can without breaking form.
You'll feel results quicker!

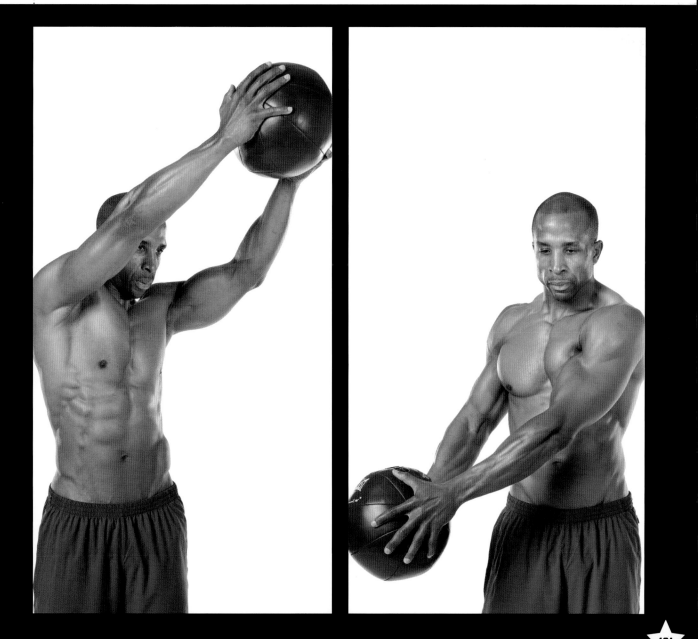

13. MEDICINE BALL WOOD CHOPPER

A great move for anyone playing a sport that requires a swinging motion such as baseball, tennis, or golf, the medicine ball wood chopper builds core strength while really amping up your cardiovascular conditioning. Try doing this movement with intensity and speed and you'll work up a sweat in no time.

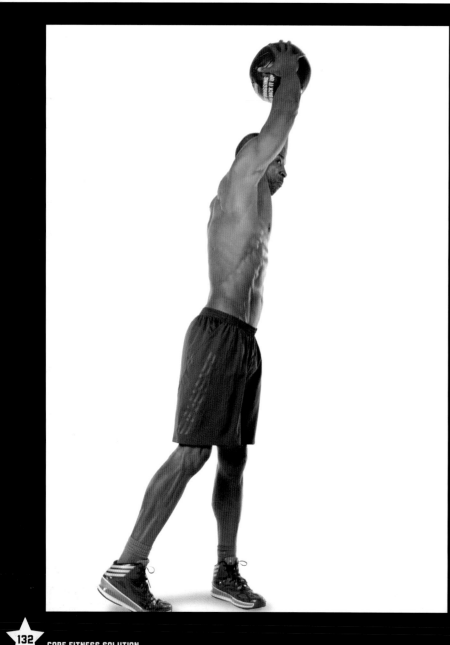

START
Stand with your feet shoulder-width apart and a slight arch in your right foot. Hold the medicine ball above you with your arms outstretched toward the ceiling as though you were about to smash the ball down on the ground.

BEGINNER

You can perform this exercise without a medicine ball to make it a little easier while you master the movement.

ADVANCED

Slam the ball down on the end of each rep to make this move a little harder. After every two reps, do a 180 degree jump turn in the direction of your downward motion.

ACTION

Thrust the ball down toward the ground and at your side, immediately return to the starting position with a slight pause and repeat the movement. Keep your feet flat on the floor and your arms outstretched.

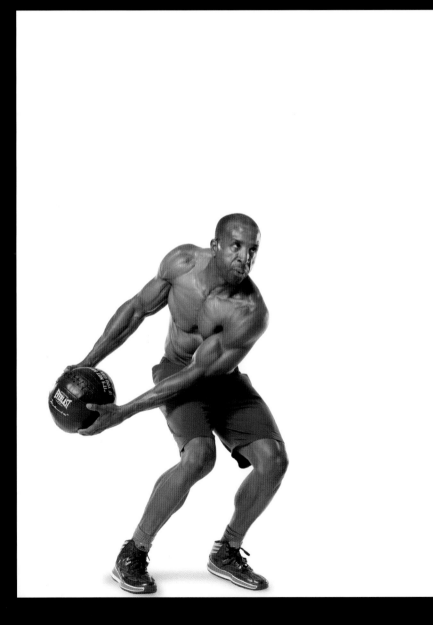

14. DECLINE MEDICINE BALL TOSS

To do the decline medicine ball toss as described here, you'll need a decline bench, a medicine ball, and a partner to throw the ball back to you. However, there are many substitutions that can be equally effective. You can lie on a flat surface or straight bench and bounce a medicine ball or basketball off the wall. Just remember to keep your body positioning as close to the original movement as possible, and focus more on the contraction than simply tossing the ball around.

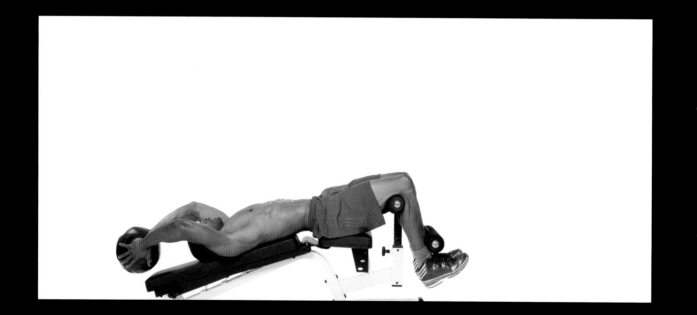

START Get onto a decline bench with your legs wrapped appropriately around the pads for your ankles and knees. Lie back with a medicine ball in your hands. Extend your arms

ACTION Crunch upward into a seated position and toss the ball at your training partner (or facing wall) while you're reaching the top of the movement. From there, your partner should throw the ball back to you as you are simultaneously returning to the starting

BEGINNER

If you want to make this move easier, try it without the ball or, simply, without the toss.

ADVANCED

Make this move a little more challenging with a heavier ball or get your partner to throw the medicine ball harder when he or she returns it on your way back to the starting position.

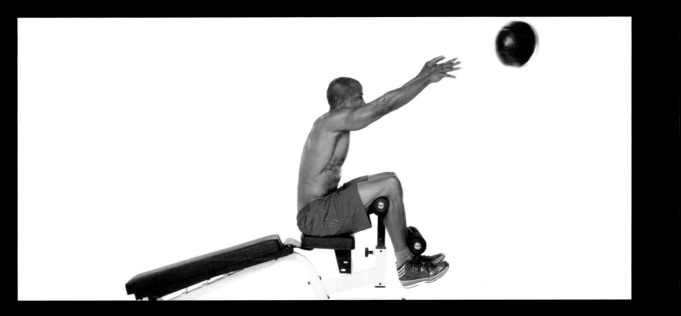

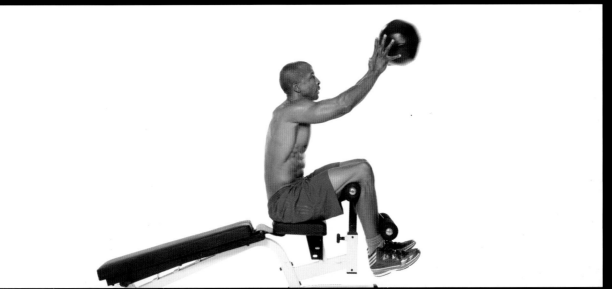

15. CORKSCREW

This is one of those moves that many people overlook or perform incorrectly. At a glance, the corkscrew may look easy or simply ineffective, but, if done properly, you'll hit virtually every angle of your core. If performed incorrectly, expect to look like a fish out of water. Focus on your form. A few reps done correctly are worth a lot more than a dozen that are not.

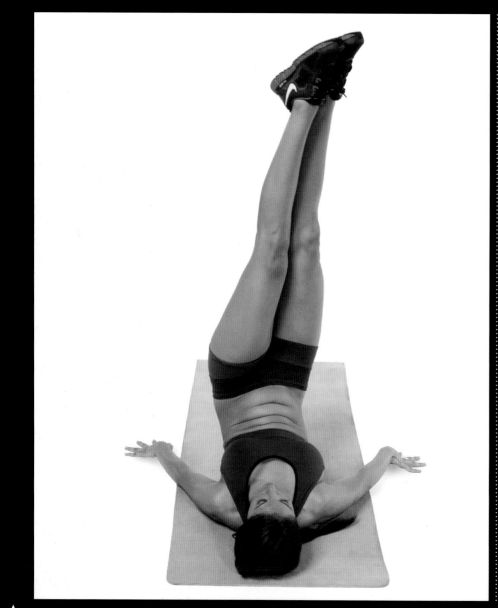

START
Lie flat on the floor with your legs pointed straight up and your heels parallel to the ceiling. Place your arms flat on the floor at your sides for balance.

BEGINNER

To make this move easier, place your hands under your back for extra balance and a slight head start on the reps.

ADVANCED

Want more out of this move? Try holding the rep for two counts at the top of the contraction. Want to take it even further? Hold a dumbbell between your feet or use ankle weights.

ACTION

Thrust your legs up while twisting your lower body. Your lower back should leave the ground in this movement. Repeat the rep so your body twists to both sides.

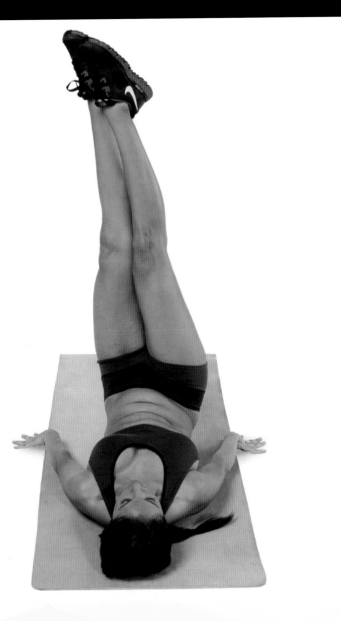

16. REVERSE HYPEREXTENSIONS

If you've done this move before, chances are you've done it wrong. Most people will bounce through each rep, extend past the point of working their core into a stretch, hug a weight plate that forces you to cheat or, worse yet, do it on the machine, which makes you most prone to injury. Just think of this as touching your toes while in the hyperextension bench. All the extras only take away from the benefits.

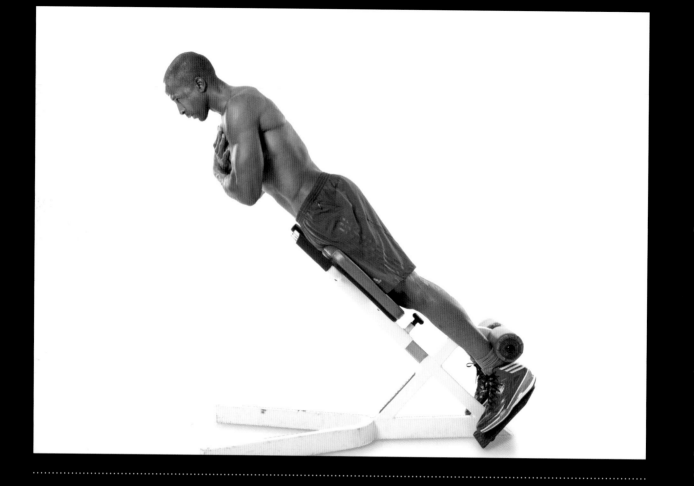

START Get onto the hyperextension bench so the front pads are at your pelvis, not your waist. Cross your arms in front of your chest.

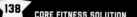

BEGINNER

If this move is too difficult for you, try doing a back stretch from the floor. Lying face down with your arms at your sides, slowly bring your upper body off the ground. Some trainers refer to this move as the prone cobra with your hands out at your sides, or the Superman exercise, with your arms straight out in front of you.

ADVANCED

You can twist to the side at the end of each rep to get more out of this movement (see photo on page 140).

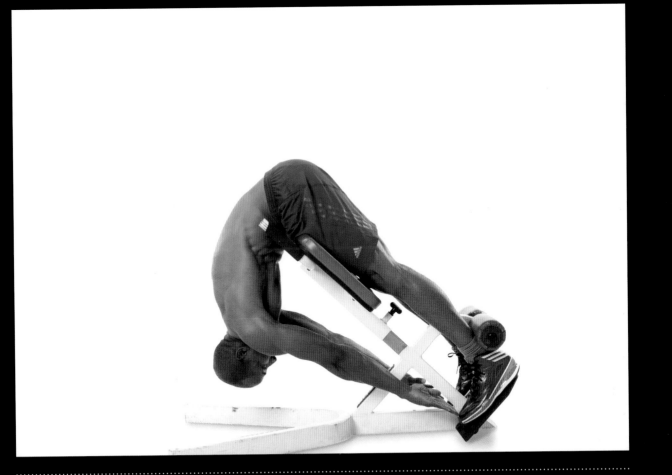

ACTION Lower your body while extending your arms, reaching for your toes. Return to the starting position.

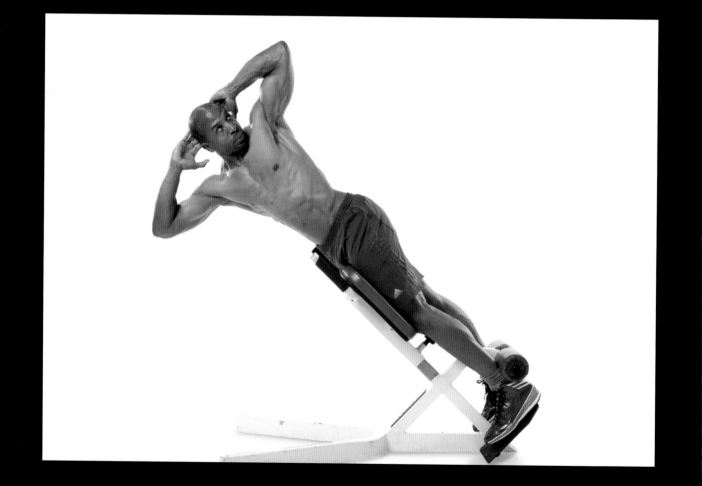

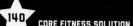

17. ISOMETRIC V-HOLD

Remember gym class warm-ups? A lot of physical education teachers had you do push-ups and sit-ups and occasionally would throw in a V-sit. What followed was a gymnasium full of kids jerking their upper bodies and legs toward each other like a faulty rollaway bed. The V-sit has its merits, but the V-hold is a move that really harnesses the most of your core.

BEGINNER
If holding the V is too difficult, put your hands in the inner bend of your knees to balance and then let go once you've found the V shape. Or perform the hold with bended knees, but do not allow your feet to touch the ground.

ADVANCED
Kick up the intensity by quickly moving your arms up and down while maintaining the proper form.

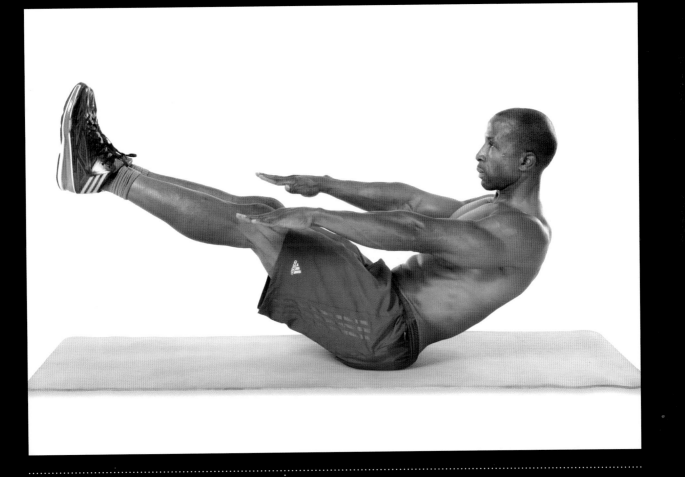

START Lie flat on the floor with your legs together and your arms at your sides.

ACTION Raise your upper body off the ground while lifting your legs up, creating a V shape with your body. Extend your arms so your forearms are parallel to the ground. Hold this position for as long as possible. Do not arch your back or hunch your shoulders forward.

18. JUMP SQUAT WITH TWIST

Not what you were expecting? Not to worry. This exercise will target your overall core, building strength and improving your stability—and the added jump will build explosiveness in your legs, which is perfect for your basketball game. Your next dunk is all the thanks we need.

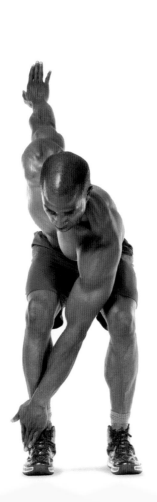

START
Stand with your feet shoulder-width apart. Squat down so your hamstrings are parallel to the ground and your left hand is touching the outside of your right ankle (alternate sides on each rep)

BEGINNER

Make this a little easier by touching the inside of your far ankle, not the outside (see photo on page 144). This will make the squat and twist easier, allowing you to focus on the contraction and the jump thereafter.

ADVANCED

If you're finding this move too easy, try spinning in the air 180 degrees so you make a half circle rotation from where you originally started. Landing mechanics is everything. Do not continue to jump if you are not landing with your feet shoulder-width apart, feet straight, and knees bent. Remember not to swing your arms to get through the spinning.

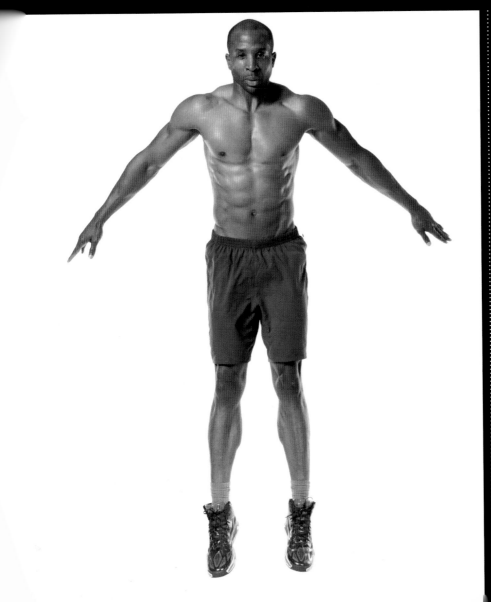

ACTION

Jump up, straightening out your torso while twisting in midair so you land facing to the right of where you started (about 90 degrees from your original jump).

FOCUS

When you're leaping into the air, don't just jump. Instead, use your core to guide your body through the explosion. It'll be moving your entire torso up into an erect position and swinging your body through the jump that was propelled by your legs.

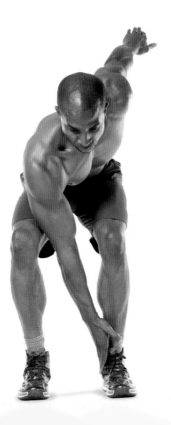

19. BRIDGE

If you ever clowned around in gym class, you've done this one already. This time you'll probably find it a lot harder than your twelve-year-old version did in years gone by.

BEGINNER
Use a Bosu ball to make it easier to get your body off the ground when doing this exercise.

ADVANCED
Hold the bridge at the top of the contraction for two counts to make this more difficult. To add even more difficulty, kick out your feet one at a time.

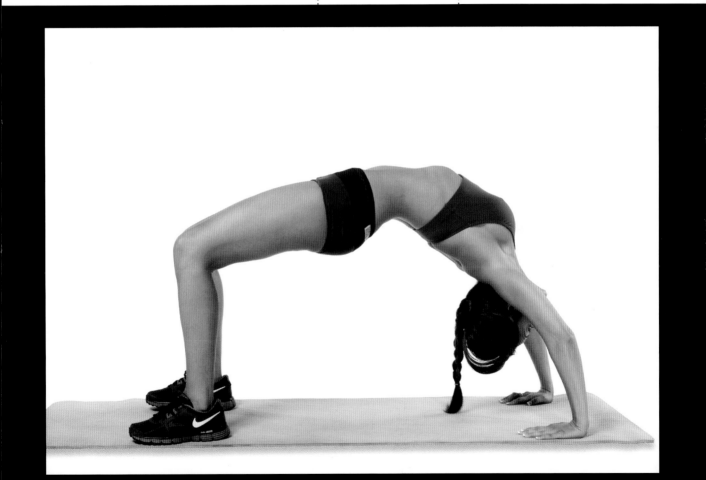

START Lie flat on the floor with your legs bent and your feet flat. Place your palms on the floor beside your head, shoulder-width apart and elbows pointed up.

ACTION Using your feet and hands for balance, thrust your body up using your core strength. Slowly lower your body to avoid injury when returning to the starting position.

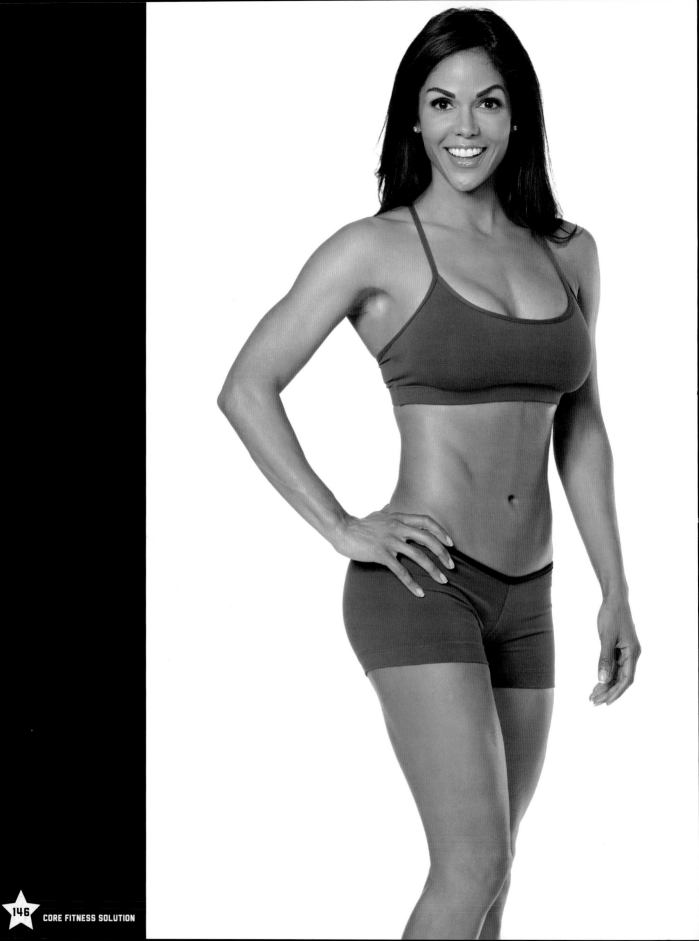

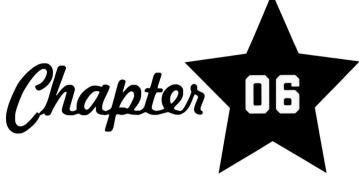

Chapter 06

CORE FITNESS SOLUTION TOTAL BODY PLAN

WHEN YOU PURCHASED THIS BOOK, IT WAS OBVIOUS THAT YOU WANTED A SOLUTION. WHILE THE PREVIOUS CHAPTERS FOCUS ON YOUR CORE, THIS CHAPTER IS DEVOTED TO ALL YOUR NON-CORE WORKOUTS AND THE HIGH-INTENSITY ACTIVITIES THAT WILL HAVE YOU HARNESSING YOUR CORE STRENGTH AND STABILITY THROUGHOUT.

First, we will walk you through some specific approaches for your total body workouts that you can perform in conjunction with your customized core plans. From there, we will give you some circuits for total body muscle growth, fat loss and cardiovascular improvement. After that, we will discuss cardio and how it fits into your solution for a better, healthier life—complete with short but effective challenge sessions for virtually any cardio activity.

Finally, this chapter will give you a combination of both cardio and total body exercises with some unique multi-exercise mini circuits that can be done anywhere and can fit into even the tightest of schedules.

YOUR WORKOUTS

As you can see from the following charts (pages 149–151), we've designed a workout plan that consists of two workouts and a legend to track your progress and increased fitness level. Within each workout are three stages, progressing in difficulty, and three categories of exercises. Your goal, much like the core workouts in the previous chapters, is to work your way through each stage. Move on to Workout 2 once you've mastered the final stage of Workout 1. Perform four circuits every workout.

RESISTANCE TRAINING

Some people just want to have a visible six-pack. Others just want to be healthier. The principles throughout this book are applicable to both, and this chapter is no different. If you want clearly defined abs, then you need to lessen your body fat. Resistance training at high intensity will yield those results. If you want to be healthier, fitter or a better athlete, or simply want to transform from overweight to average, then high-intensity resistance training has to be in your regime as well. These workouts achieve results because they test your limits on all planes of motion and are based on the high-intensity interval training and muscle confusion principles, which are proven results-generating philosophies for any fitness level.

HIGH-INTENSITY INTERVAL TRAINING

Think of high-intensity interval training (HIIT) as the elite form of interval training. Far beyond just timed intervals of exercise or cardio, HIIT combines short, intense workout periods with less demanding recovery exercises. This is a workout philosophy that will keep your heart rate elevated and will also test your muscular endurance. Because intense exercise is relative, the more demanding intervals of a session can last anywhere from 10 seconds to 3 minutes—it all depends on your fitness level, and only you can judge it while you're actually doing it.

DURATION AND INTENSITY LEVELS

LEVEL	DURATION OF CIRCUIT (MIN/SEC)	TOTAL TIME* (MIN/SEC)
BEGINNER (15 seconds per exercise)	1:00 circuit followed by 1:00 rest	8:00
INTERMEDIATE (20 seconds per exercise)	1:20 circuit followed by 1:00 rest	9:20
AVERAGE (25 seconds per exercise)	1:40 circuit followed by 1:00 rest	10:40
ADVANCED (30 seconds per exercise)	2 :00 circuit followed by 1:00 rest	12:00
SUPERIOR (45 seconds per exercise)	Each exercise is followed by 0:15 rest. Each circuit is followed by 2 :00 rest.	24:00
ELITE (60 seconds per exercise)	Each exercise is followed by 0:20 second rest. Each circuit is followed by 2:00 rest.	28:00

Perform each circuit 4 times.

WORKOUT 1

	STAGE 1	STAGE 2	STAGE 2
SQUATS	Squat or air squat	Cross-legged jump squat	Squat and curl with resistance bands or dumbbells
PUSH-UPS	Push-up on knees or wall push-up	Push-up	Push-up with alternating leg extension
LUNGES	Stationary lunge (2 circuits for each leg)	Walking lunge	Jumping lunge
PRONE RETRACTIONS	I-Y-T-W*	I-Y-T-W*	I-Y-T-W*

*Do a different letter for each circuit.

MUSCLE CONFUSION

Muscle confusion is a very simple concept. When you train the same way for too long—using the same exercises, sets, reps, and intensity—your body gets used to the work you're making it do and results begin to taper off. Bottom line: You do something enough times, it becomes common and no longer challenging. Muscle confusion takes this principle and forces change within your workout philosophy—different exercises, sets and reps, for example—to ensure that your body is always being tested and working at optimum capacity.

WORKOUT 2

	STAGE 1	STAGE 2	STAGE 2
SPEED SKATERS	Stepping speed skater (with hand to foot)	Speed skater (with hand to foot and back leg landing)	Advanced speed skater with only front leg landing (may add medicine ball)
PUSH-UPS	Walk out push-up on knees (2 reps at each walkout)	Walk out push-up	Renegade walk out push-up (with alternate row)
LUNGES	Stationary lunge with twist (2 circuits for each leg)	Walking lunge with twist	Walking lunge with twist and press
SINGLE LEG DEADLIFTS (2 circuits for each leg)	Assisted single leg deadlift	Single leg deadlift	Single leg deadlift with weight

HOW TO DO THE MOVES IN WORKOUT 1

SQUATS

With your feet shoulder-width apart and a relaxed stance in your knees, drop your butt down to the floor until your hamstrings are parallel to the ground.

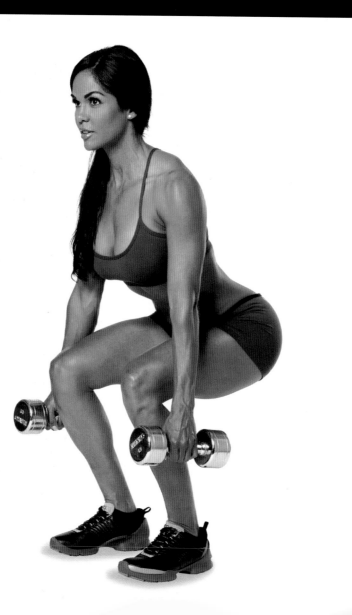

VARIATIONS

Air squat: Perform this as previously described, but go up to the balls of your feet when returning to a standing position.

Cross-legged jump squat: Starting in a squat position, jump up and land with your legs crossed, quickly bouncing from the balls of your feet back out into a squat position.

Squat and curl: Perform a squat and curl two dumbbells or resistance bands after returning to a standing position.

PUSH-UPS

Lie on the ground, making a straight line
of your body, balancing yourself on your
hands and toes. Press up so your arms are
straight and return to the starting position.

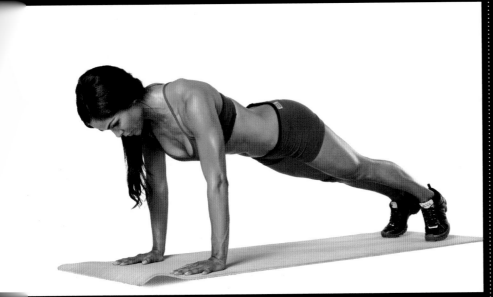

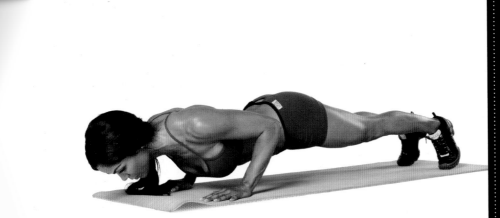

VARIATIONS

Push-up on knees: Get
into a typical push-up
position, but rest your
weight on your knees
throughout the reps.

Wall push-up: Perform a
push-up from a standing
position, facing a wall.

**Push-up with
alternating leg
extension:** Perform
the reps while lifting
one leg off the ground,
alternating legs with
each rep.

LUNGES

Stationary lunge: Stand with your feet shoulder-width apart. Step forward with one leg and bend forward on your knee until your forward leg's hamstring makes a 90-degree angle with the floor. Your trailing leg is straight and making a 45-degree angle with the floor.

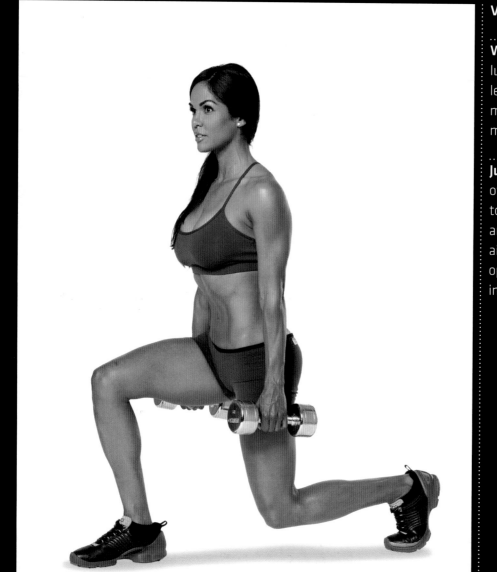

VARIATIONS

Walking lunge: Perform lunges, alternating legs on each rep so you move forward with each movement.

Jumping lunge: Instead of just stepping forward to lunge, jump up and switch legs in the air, landing with the opposite leg forward and in a lunge position.

PRONE RETRACTION

With letter shapes: I, Y, T, and W: Lie face down with your toes pointed down to the floor. Squeeze your quads and glutes, which will cause your knees to lift off of the floor. While keeping a neutral spine and your head down facing the floor, lift your arms in an I-Y-T and squeeze into a W. Hold each position for 2 seconds. After the W, relax for two seconds and repeat.

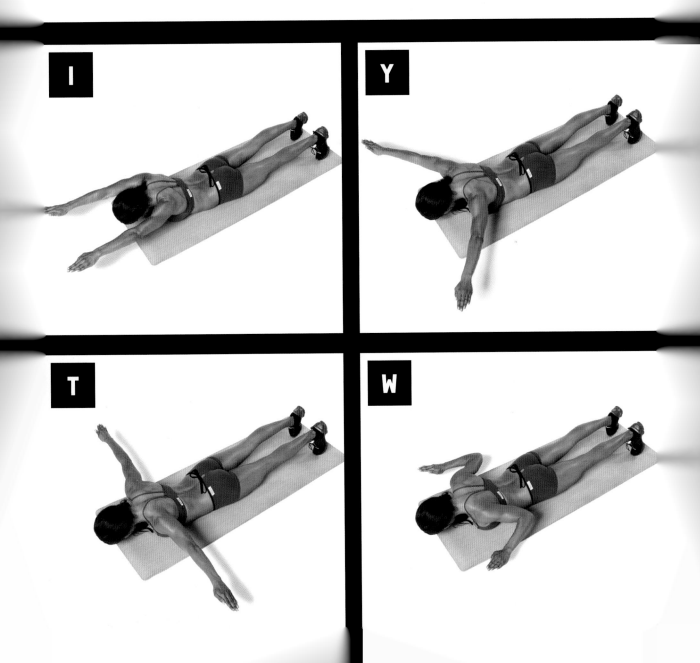

HOW TO DO THE MOVES IN WORKOUT 2

SPEED SKATERS

Mimicking the stride of an ice hockey player, stand with your feet shoulder-width apart and leap side to side, landing on alternating legs for each rep.

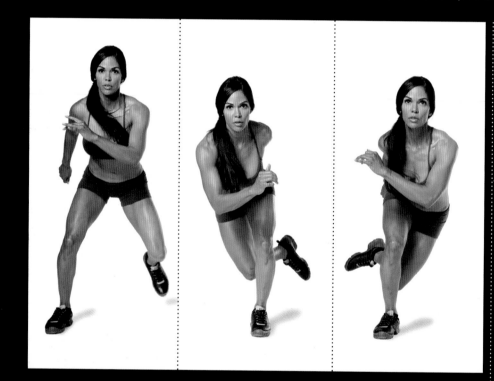

VARIATIONS

Stepping speed skater: This is similar to the speed skater, but do not leave the ground and rely on more of a shuffle to complete each rep. Touch your front foot with your opposite hand with your chest and head up, looking forward.

Advanced speed skater: Land only on your front leg and possibly hold a weight throughout your sets.

PUSH-UPS

Walk out push-up: Perform a typical push-up and stride forward on your hands, alternating over two reps (so each hand is responsible for a stride forward). Return to a standing position, then back into a push-up to perform another set of two.

LUNGES

Stationary (and walking) lunge with twist: Perform as previously directed in Workout 1, but add in a torso twist at the end of each rep.

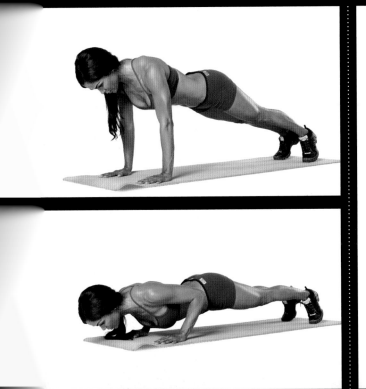

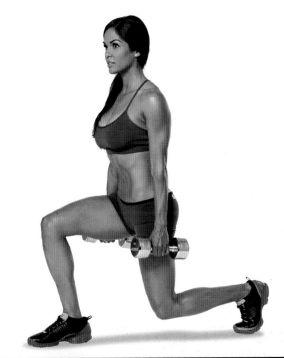

VARIATIONS

Walk out push-up on knees: As described above, but balance your weight on your knees.

Renegade walk out push-up: This is similar to the walk out push-up, but add an arm row after each forward stride.

VARIATIONS

Walking lunge with twist and press: Perform this move as previously described, but press up the weight you are holding after the twist.

SINGLE LEG DEADLIFTS

Kicking back one leg, bend forward, creating a straight line with your torso and trailing leg. The arm on the side with your leg up falls in front of you. Repeat for both legs.

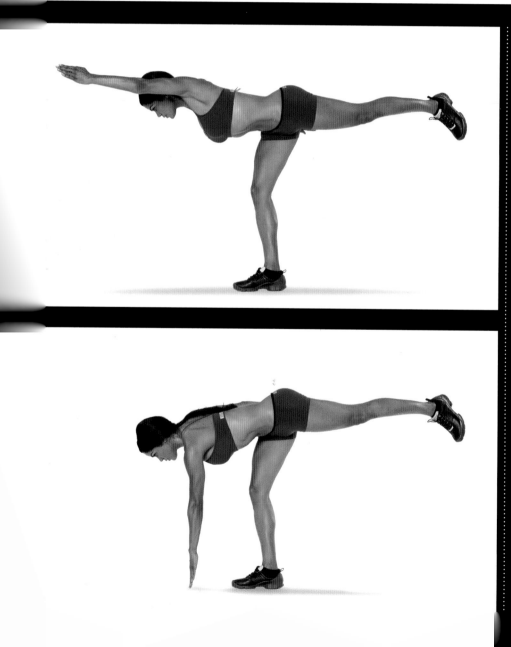

VARIATIONS

Assisted single leg deadlift: Perform a typical single leg deadlift, but brace yourself on either side to ensure you don't fall.

Single leg deadlift with weight: Perform the single leg deadlift with a dumbbell in the hand on the side of the trailing leg.

YOUR CARDIO PLAN

The basis of this cardio plan is that you can perform this challenge while doing just about any timed cardiovascular activity, as long as you can maintain the intensity level dictated by the chart that follows. If the following cardio session is too demanding for you, do steady-state cardio for 45 minutes to an hour, but try to include some sprints in each session so you can grow accustomed to the intensity and eventually graduate to the following plan.

INTENSITY	DURATION
SPRINT (Fast; High Intensity)	1 minute
JOG (Slow; Low Intensity)	2 minutes

Note: On days that you're doing resistance training, perform 10 rounds of this interval (maxing out at 30 minutes). Do 15 rounds (maxing out at 45 minutes) if you're only doing cardio on the day of training.

YOUR TOTAL BODY QUICK FIX 1

1. DEADLIFT → 2. ROW → 3. KICKBACK → 4. JUMP

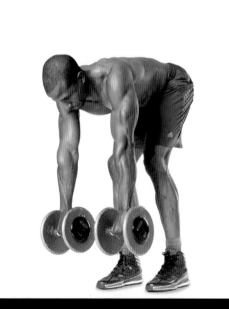

DEADLIFT

Holding two dumbbells, bend forward with a slight bend in your knees without arching or hunching your back.

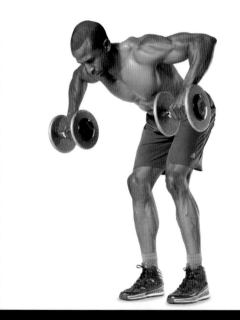

ROW

Pull the dumbbells back so you create a 90-degree angle with your elbows

If you find yourself short on time and can't seem to get through the workouts listed in this chapter, this section offers you two quick fixes. These are by no means intended to replace the workouts previously detailed, but if you really can't get your workout in, performing one of these mini-circuits will keep you on track. Execution is really quite simple: Pick one of the two following quick fixes and perform them to failure without resting periods and at your highest intensity level. This means you're moving quickly, with purpose, with good form and with focus on getting the most out of every single nuance of each step.

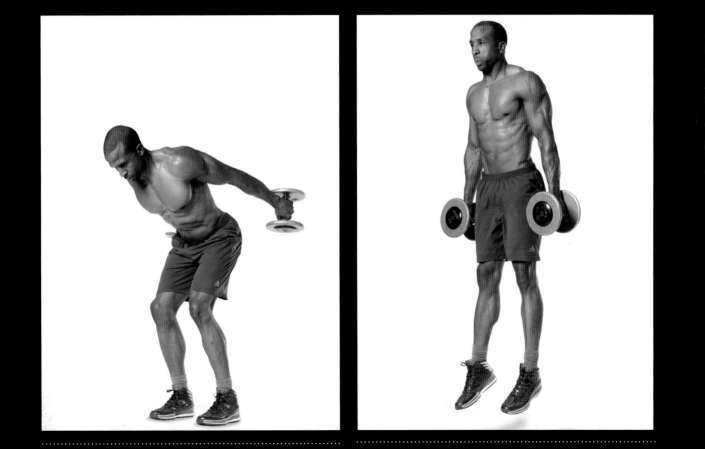

KICKBACK

Kick the weights back so your arms are straight.

JUMP

Jump up while allowing your arms to come to your sides.

YOUR TOTAL BODY QUICK FIX 2

1. SQUAT → 2. LUNGE → 3. HAMMER CURL → 4. SHOULDER PRESS

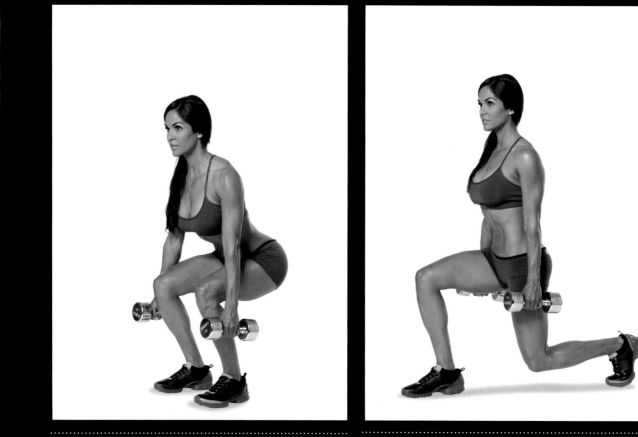

SQUAT

Holding two dumbbells, squat down so your hamstrings are almost parallel to the floor and you have a slight arch in your lower back.

LUNGE

Lunge forward on one leg. Your trailing leg is bent at the knee and your knee is just off the ground.

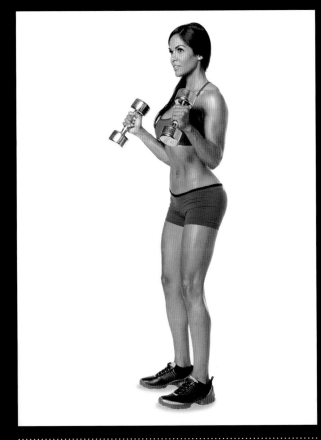

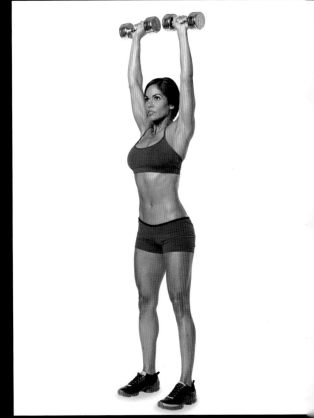

HAMMER CURL

Return to a standing position and curl the
weights up without twisting your wrists.

SHOULDER PRESS

Press the weights up with the palms of
your hands facing outward.

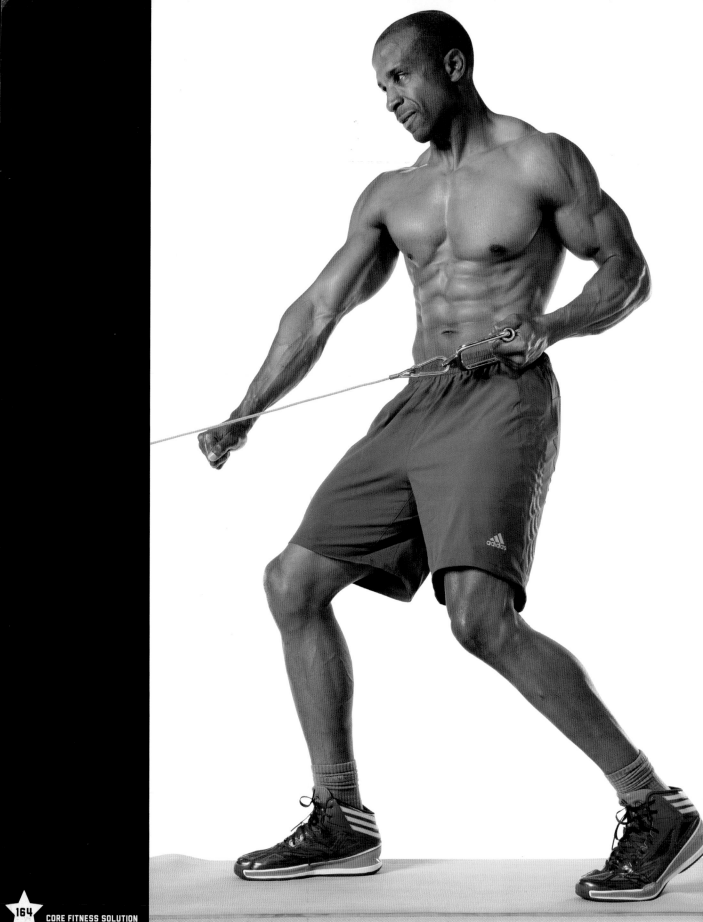

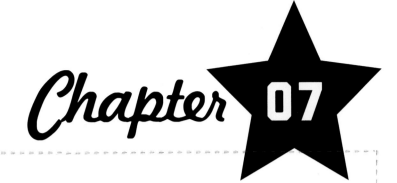

Chapter 07

YOUR TRAINING LOG

AS YOU PROGRESS THROUGH YOUR CUSTOMIZED CORE WORKOUT, WE ENCOURAGE YOU TO TRACK YOUR PROGRESS IN THE FOLLOWING PAGES.

Core STRENGTH SOLUTION
TRAINING LOGS

**CORE FITNESS SOLUTION
WORKOUT LOG (SAMPLE)**

DATE:

EXERCISE	REPS
LOWER ABS 1: *Flutter Kicks*	18
LOWER ABS 2: *Hanging Leg Raise*	10
UPPER ABS 1: *Stability Ball Crunch*	15
UPPER ABS 2: *Dead Bug*	9
OBLIQUES 1: *Side Plank*	18
OBLIQUES 2: *Seated Broom Twist*	38
TOTAL CORE 1: *Mountain Climbers*	24
TOTAL CORE 2: *Isometric V-Hold*	22

DATE:

EXERCISE	REPS
LOWER ABS 1:	
LOWER ABS 2:	
UPPER ABS 1:	
UPPER ABS 2:	
OBLIQUES 1:	
OBLIQUES 2:	
TOTAL CORE 1:	
TOTAL CORE 2:	

DATE:

EXERCISE	REPS
LOWER ABS 1:	
LOWER ABS 2:	
UPPER ABS 1:	
UPPER ABS 2:	
OBLIQUES 1:	
OBLIQUES 2:	
TOTAL CORE 1:	
TOTAL CORE 2:	

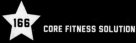

DATE:

EXERCISE	REPS
LOWER ABS 1:	
LOWER ABS 2:	
UPPER ABS 1:	
UPPER ABS 2:	
OBLIQUES 1:	
OBLIQUES 2:	
TOTAL CORE 1:	
TOTAL CORE 2:	

DATE:

EXERCISE	REPS
LOWER ABS 1:	
LOWER ABS 2:	
UPPER ABS 1:	
UPPER ABS 2:	
OBLIQUES 1:	
OBLIQUES 2:	
TOTAL CORE 1:	
TOTAL CORE 2:	

DATE:

EXERCISE	REPS
LOWER ABS 1:	
LOWER ABS 2:	
UPPER ABS 1:	
UPPER ABS 2:	
OBLIQUES 1:	
OBLIQUES 2:	
TOTAL CORE 1:	
TOTAL CORE 2:	

Core STRENGTH SOLUTION TRAINING LOGS

CORE FITNESS SOLUTION
WORKOUT LOG

DATE:

EXERCISE	REPS
LOWER ABS 1:	
LOWER ABS 2:	
UPPER ABS 1:	
UPPER ABS 2:	
OBLIQUES 1:	
OBLIQUES 2:	
TOTAL CORE 1:	
TOTAL CORE 2:	

DATE:

EXERCISE	REPS
LOWER ABS 1:	
LOWER ABS 2:	
UPPER ABS 1:	
UPPER ABS 2:	
OBLIQUES 1:	
OBLIQUES 2:	
TOTAL CORE 1:	
TOTAL CORE 2:	

DATE:

EXERCISE	REPS
LOWER ABS 1:	
LOWER ABS 2:	
UPPER ABS 1:	
UPPER ABS 2:	
OBLIQUES 1:	
OBLIQUES 2:	
TOTAL CORE 1:	
TOTAL CORE 2:	

DATE:

EXERCISE	REPS
LOWER ABS 1:	
LOWER ABS 2:	
UPPER ABS 1:	
UPPER ABS 2:	
OBLIQUES 1:	
OBLIQUES 2:	
TOTAL CORE 1:	
TOTAL CORE 2:	

DATE:

EXERCISE	REPS
LOWER ABS 1:	
LOWER ABS 2:	
UPPER ABS 1:	
UPPER ABS 2:	
OBLIQUES 1:	
OBLIQUES 2:	
TOTAL CORE 1:	
TOTAL CORE 2:	

DATE:

EXERCISE	REPS
LOWER ABS 1:	
LOWER ABS 2:	
UPPER ABS 1:	
UPPER ABS 2:	
OBLIQUES 1:	
OBLIQUES 2:	
TOTAL CORE 1:	
TOTAL CORE 2:	

ACKNOWLEDGMENTS

There are many people we would like to thank for making this book possible. First and foremost, we want to thank our families and God for being our strength and for always driving us to do better. We would also like to thank the tireless efforts of our publishing house and the amazing staff including Jessica, John, Katie, David, and everyone else who helped bring our ideas to the page and, ultimately, to you.

A special thanks to Amber Day, our cover girl and interior model, Talia Terese, who is also featured in our workouts, and to photographer Robert Reiff, who shot all of this book at MagicLight studios in Los Angeles.

There are many more folks who deserve a thanks but none more than the following special people: Youla, Tom, James, Lisa, Edwina, Cherise, Danielle, Aisha, Veda, Masaun, Isaiah, Ellis, Natalie, Jackie, Danielle C, Kelly, and all of our wonderful clients, fitness friends and associates.

Special thanks to Elisabetta Rogiani (www.rogiani.com) for the female fashions shot in this book and to Nancy Jambazian for hair and makeup.

We want to dedicate this book to anyone who has ever given up on themselves or have been told that they could not achieve greatness. This book is for anyone who wants to be their best. Last but not least, thank you for buying this book and making our vision a part of your life!

ABOUT THE AUTHORS

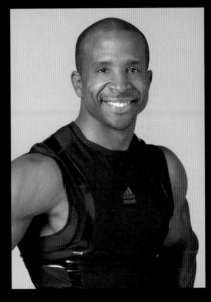

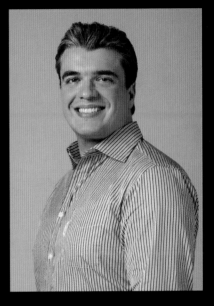

KENDALL WOOD, NASM, C.P.T., M.Ed., the "King of Abs," is a multi-time fitness magazine cover model, NASM–certified personal trainer, health advocate, and a forerunner in the fight against childhood obesity. His foundation, Smart Moves, works to end obesity for children by partnering up with school boards and family associations. He is also the promoter of FitScience's annual fitness contest in Atlanta.

MICHAEL DE MEDEIROS is the former vice president and editor in chief of *Men's Fitness* magazine, former editor-in-chief of *Maximum Fitness* magazine, and author of 13 books, including historical biographies, educational textbooks, and active health and fitness books. He has been nominated and shortlisted for several awards, including best book and best book in a series (Weigl Publishers).

INDEX

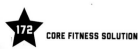

CHECK OUT THESE OTHER FAIR WINDS PRESS FITNESS TITLES!

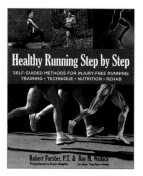

Healthy Running Step by Step
Robert Forster and Roy Wallack
ISBN: 978-1-59233-605-0

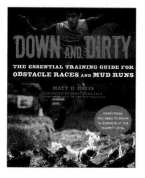

Down and Dirty
Matt Davis
ISBN: 978-1-59233-599-2

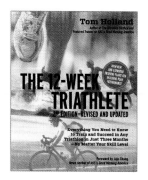

The 12-Week Triathlete, Second Edition
Tom Holland
ISBN: 978-1-59233-458-2

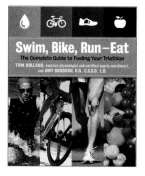

Swim, Bike, Run, Eat
Tom Holland and Amy Goodson
ISBN: 978-1-59233-606-7

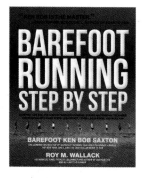

Barefoot Running Step by Step
Roy Wallack and Ken Saxton
ISBN: 978-1-59233-465-0

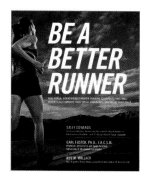

Be a Better Runner
Sally Edwards, Carl Foster, and Roy Wallack
ISBN: 978-1-59233-424-7

FAIR WINDS
P R E S S
Available online or at your local book store.
www.fairwindspress.com

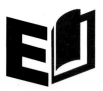

Our books are available as E-Books, too!
Many of our bestselling titles are now available as E-Books.
Visit www.Qbookshop.com to find links to e-vendors!